NURSING ASSISTANT/ NURSE AIDE

FLASH REVIEW

NURSING ASSISTANT/ NURSE AIDE

FLASH REVIEW

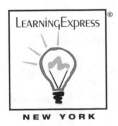

LEARNINGEXPRESS®

NEW YORK

Cataloging-in-Publication Data is on file with the Library of Congress.

Printed in the United States of America

9 8 7 6 5 4 3 2 1

First Edition

ISBN 978-1-57685-951-3

For more information or to place an order, contact LearningExpress at:
    80 Broad Street
    4th Floor
    New York, NY 10004

CONTENTS

INTRODUCTION

Welcome to the healthcare profession!

As a nursing assistant/nurse aide, you will be a critical member of the healthcare team, regardless of whether you work for a hospital, rehabilitation center, long-term care facility, home care agency, or other healthcare facility. Preparing for your certification exam is an important rite of passage to your new career.

About the NNAAP Exam

The National Nurse Aide Assessment Program (NNAAP), which is owned by the National Council of State Boards of Nursing (NCSBN), is the largest nurse aide certification examination program in the United States. The NNAAP contains two components—a written or oral examination and a skills demonstration. Candidates must pass both components before they can be added to their state nurse aide registry.

As of this writing, 25 NCSBN jurisdictions use the NNAAP exam to determine nurse aide competency. Therefore, you should check with your state agency to find the requirements in your state.

About This Book

This book contains more than 600 concepts, terms, and skills to help prepare you for the NNAAP exam. These are divided into six parts: (1) Terminology, (2) Body Systems, (3) Human Needs, (4) The Nursing Assistant Role, (5) Nursing Assistant Skills, and (6) Nursing Assistant Care of Special Populations. Each of these parts is broken down into specific sections that contain the concepts, terms, and skills. Each page contains one to three concepts, terms, and skills on the front, with the description of each on the back.

The term *nursing assistant* is used throughout the book for consistency, as is the term *client*. *Nursing assistant* is synonymous with *nurse aide*. *Client* is used here as a general term for consistency, even though the persons cared for by nursing assistants are usually called *patients* in hospital settings, *residents* in long-term care and rehabilitation settings, and *clients* in home care.

How to Use This Book

This book is not a substitute for your textbook. It is designed to be part of your study plan.

The information presented here is pretty comprehensive, so please do not try to read this book in one sitting or try to memorize all the information. Instead, set aside about 30 minutes each day to review the book. Since the book is portable, carry it with you so you can review a few pages when you find yourself with some free time, like when waiting in line at the grocery store. Quiz yourself periodically, and mark off the pages as you master them.

Good luck on your NNAAP study plan and exam!

Terminology

ROOT WORDS, PREFIXES, AND SUFFIXES THAT BEGIN WITH A

. . . .

ROOT WORDS, PREFIXES, AND SUFFIXES THAT BEGIN WITH B

. . . .

ROOT WORDS, PREFIXES, AND SUFFIXES THAT BEGIN WITH C

Root/Prefix/Suffix	Meaning	Example
a-, an-	not or without	aseptic, analgesic
ab-	away	abduction
ad-	toward	adduction
angi(o)-	blood vessel	angiogram
ante-	before	anteroom
anti-	against	antibody, antipsychotic

Root/Prefix/Suffix	Meaning	Example
bi-	two	bifocal
brady-	slow	bradycardia
bronch-	bronchus	bronchitis

Root/Prefix/Suffix	Meaning	Example
carcin(o)-	cancer	carcinoma
cardi(o)-	pertaining to the heart	cardiology
circum-	around	circumcision
cirrho-	red or orange	cirrhosis
co-	with or together	coagulate
contra-	against	contraindicate
cyan(o)-	denoting a blue color	cyanosis
cyst(o)-, cyst(i)-	pertaining to the urinary bladder	cystoscopy

ROOT WORDS, PREFIXES, AND SUFFIXES THAT BEGIN WITH D

. . . .

ROOT WORDS, PREFIXES, AND SUFFIXES THAT BEGIN WITH E

. . . .

ROOT WORDS, PREFIXES, AND SUFFIXES THAT BEGIN WITH G

Root/Prefix/Suffix	Meaning	Example
dent-	pertaining to teeth	dentist
dermat(o)-, derm(o)-	pertaining to the skin	dermatology
dextr(o)-	right (side)	dextrocardia
di-	two	diplopia
dia-	apart, separation	diaphragm
dia-	throughout	diabetes
-dipsia	thirst	polydipsia
dys-	bad, difficult	dyspepsia

. . . .

Root/Prefix/Suffix	Meaning	Example
-ectomy	removal of a body part	hysterectomy
-edema	swelling	myxedema
-emesis	vomiting	hematemesis
-emia	blood condition	anemia
erythr(o)-	red	erythrocyte
eu-	true, good, well, new	euphoric
ex-	out of, away from	excision
extra-	outside	extrauterine

. . . .

Root/Prefix/Suffix	Meaning	Example
gastr(o)-	pertaining to the stomach	gastritis
gingiv-	pertaining to the gums	gingivitis
gloss-	pertaining to the tongue	glossitis
-graphy	process of recording	angiography
gyn-	Pertaining to female reproductive organ	gynecologist

ROOT WORDS, PREFIXES, AND SUFFIXES THAT BEGIN WITH H

. . . .

ROOT WORDS, PREFIXES, AND SUFFIXES THAT BEGIN WITH I

. . . .

ROOT WORDS, PREFIXES, AND SUFFIXES THAT BEGIN WITH L

Root/Prefix/Suffix	Meaning	Example
hem(o)-,	pertaining to blood	hemophilia
hemi-	half	hemiplegia
hepat-	pertaining to the liver	hepatitis
heter(o)-	different	heterosexual
hom(o)-	the same	homosexual
hydr(o)-	water	hydrocephalus
hyper-	above normal	hypertension
hyp(o)-	below normal	hypotension
hyster(o)-	pertaining to the uterus	hysterectomy

Root/Prefix/Suffix	Meaning	Example
in-	not	inorganic
in-	within	infect
inter-	between, among	interdisciplinary
intra-	within	intradisciplinary
-ism	condition, disease	hypothyroidism
iso-	equal	isotonic
-itis	inflammation	tonsillitis

Root/Prefix/Suffix	Meaning	Example
leuc-, leuk-	white	leukemia
Lip(o)-	fat	liposuction
-logist	specialist in a certain field	pathologist
-logy	study or practice of a certain field	hematology
lymph(o)-	lymph, pertaining to fluid in nodes, vessels	lymphedema

ROOT WORDS, PREFIXES, AND SUFFIXES THAT BEGIN WITH M

. . . .

ROOT WORDS, PREFIXES, AND SUFFIXES THAT BEGIN WITH N

. . . .

ROOT WORDS, PREFIXES, AND SUFFIXES THAT BEGIN WITH O

Root/Prefix/Suffix	Meaning	Example
macr(o)-	large, long	macroscopic
mamm(o)-	breast	mammogram
melan(o)-	black, dark	melanin
mening(o)-	spinal cord	meningitis
meta-	after, behind	metacarpus
micr(o)-	small	microscope

Root/Prefix/Suffix	Meaning	Example
nas(o)-	nose	nasal
necr(o)-	death	necrosis
neo-	new	neoplasm
nephr(o)-	kidney	nephrology
nerv-	nerve	nervous
neur(o)-	nervous system	neurosurgeon

Root/Prefix/Suffix	Meaning	Example
ocul(o)-	eye	ocular
ophthalm(o)-	eye	ophthalmology
oste(o)-	bone	osteoporosis
ot(o)-	pertaining to the ear	otoscope

ROOT WORDS, PREFIXES, AND SUFFIXES THAT BEGIN WITH P

. . . .

ROOT WORDS, PREFIXES, AND SUFFIXES THAT BEGIN WITH Q

. . . .

ROOT WORDS, PREFIXES, AND SUFFIXES THAT BEGIN WITH R

Root/Prefix/Suffix	Meaning	Example
ped-, -ped	foot	pedoscope, maxilleped
pedia-	child	pediatrics
pharmaco-	medication	pharmacology
-phobia	inflated fear	acrophobia
pneum(o)-	lungs	pneumonia
poly-	many	polydipsia
post-	after	postmortem
pre-	before	prematurity
presby-	old age	presbyopia
pseud(o)-	false or fake	pseudopregnancy
psych-	the mind	psychology

Root/Prefix/Suffix	Meaning	Example
quad-	four	quadriceps

Root/Prefix/Suffix	Meaning	Example
re-	again, backward	relapse
ren(o)-	kidney	renal
rhin(o)-	nose	rhinoplasty

ROOT WORDS, PREFIXES, AND SUFFIXES THAT BEGIN WITH S

. . . .

ROOT WORDS, PREFIXES, AND SUFFIXES THAT BEGIN WITH T

. . . .

ROOT WORDS, PREFIXES, AND SUFFIXES THAT BEGIN WITH U

Root/Prefix/Suffix	Meaning	Example
-scope	instrument for viewing	stethoscope
semi-	half	seminormal
sub-	under	sublingual
super-	in excess, above	superego
supra-	above	suprasternal

Root/Prefix/Suffix	Meaning	Example
tachy-	fast	tachycardia
therm(o)-	heat	thermometer
thromb(o)-	clotting of blood	thrombus
-tomy	incision	tracheotomy
trans-	across or through	transfusion
tri-	three	triangle

Root/Prefix/Suffix	Meaning	Example
ultra-	beyond, excessive	ultrasound
un(i)-	one	uniform
ur(o)-	pertaining to urine	urology
uter(o)-	pertaining to the uterus	uterine

Nursing Assistant/Nurse Aide Flash Review

ROOT WORDS, PREFIXES, AND SUFFIXES THAT BEGIN WITH V

. . . .

Prefix or suffix	Meaning	Examples
vas(o)-	blood vessel	vasoconstriction
ven(i),- ven(o)	vein	venipuncture
-version	turning	anteversion, retroversion
vesic(o)-	bladder	vesicoureteral
viscer(o)-	internal organs	visceral

ABBREVIATIONS THAT BEGIN WITH A AND B

. . . .

ABBREVIATIONS THAT BEGIN WITH C

. . . .

Abbreviation	Meaning
ac	before meals (*ante cibum*)
ADL	activities of daily living
ad lib	as desired (*ad libitum*)
AIDS	acquired immunodeficiency syndrome
ASAP	as soon as possible
bid	twice a day (*bis in die*)
BM	bowel movement
BP	blood pressure
BR	bed rest
BPR	bathroom privileges
Bx	biopsy

Abbreviation	Meaning
C	centigrade or Celsius
CA	cancer
CBC	complete blood count
CBR	complete bed rest
CCU	coronary care unit
CHD	coronary heart disease
CHF	congestive heart failure
CNA	certified nurse aide
c/o	complains of
COPD	chronic obstructive pulmonary disease
CPR	cardiopulmonary resuscitation
CVA	cerebral vascular accident

Nursing Assistant/Nurse Aide Flash Review

ABBREVIATIONS THAT BEGIN WITH D AND E

....

ABBREVIATIONS THAT BEGIN WITH F AND G

....

Abbreviation	Meaning
d/c	discontinue
DM	diabetes mellitus
DNR	Do not resuscitate
DOA	dead on arrival
DOB	date of birth
DON	director of nursing
Dx	diagnosis
ECG or EKG	electrocardiogram
EEG	electroencephalogram
ER	emergency room

Abbreviation	Meaning
F	Fahrenheit
FBS	fasting blood sugar
fl	fluid
ft	foot
f/u	follow up
FUO	fever of unknown origin
Fx	fracture
gal	gallon
GB	gallbladder
GERD	gastroesophageal reflux disease
GSW	gunshot wound
GU	genitourinary
gyn	gynecology

Nursing Assistant/Nurse Aide Flash Review

ABBREVIATIONS THAT BEGIN WITH H AND I

. . . .

ABBREVIATIONS THAT BEGIN WITH L

. . . .

Abbreviation	Meaning
HHA	home health aide; home health agency
H$_2$O	water
HS	hour of sleep
ht or hgt (per agency policy)	height
ICU	intensive care unit
IDDM	insulin-dependent diabetes mellitus
in	inch
I&O	intake and output
IV	intravenous

Abbreviation	Meaning
lab	laboratory
liq	liquid
LLQ	left lower quadrant
LMP	last menstrual period
LP	lumbar puncture
LPN	licensed practical nurse
LRQ	lower right quadrant
LUQ	left upper quadrant
LVN	licensed vocational nurse

Nursing Assistant/Nurse Aide Flash Review

ABBREVIATIONS THAT BEGIN WITH M AND N

. . . .

ABBREVIATIONS THAT BEGIN WITH O

. . . .

Abbreviation	Meaning
max	maximum
MD	medical doctor
meds	medications
MI	myocardial infarction
mod	moderate
NA	nursing assistant
neg	negative
NG	nasogastric
NIDDM	non-insulin-dependent diabetes mellitus
norm	normal
NPO	nothing by mouth (*nil per os*)
NSAID	nonsteroidal anti-inflammatory drug
nsg	nursing
N&V	nausea and vomiting

Abbreviation	Meaning
O_2	oxygen
OA	osteoarthritis
ob	obstetrics
OJ	orange juice
OOB	out of bed
OR	operating room
ortho	orthopedics
OT	occupational therapy
oz	ounce

Nursing Assistant/Nurse Aide Flash Review

ABBREVIATIONS THAT BEGIN WITH P

....

ABBREVIATIONS THAT BEGIN WITH Q

....

Abbreviation	Meaning
p̄	after
PA	physician assistant
pap	pap smear
p̄c	after meals
PE	physical exam or pulmonary embolism
peds	pediatrics
per	by
P.M.	afternoon or evening
PM	postmortem
PO	by mouth (*per os*)
postop	postoperative
preop	preoperative
prep	preparation
prn	as needed (*pro re nata*)
PT	physical therapy

Abbreviation	Meaning
q	every (*quaque*)
qd	every day (*quaque die*)
qh	every hour (*quaque hora*)
q2h, q3h, q4h, etc.	every two hours, every three hours, every four hours, etc.
qhs	every night (*quaque hora somni*)
qid	four times a day (*quarter in die*)
qt	quart
quad	quadriplegic

Nursing Assistant/Nurse Aide Flash Review

ABBREVIATIONS THAT BEGIN WITH R

. . . .

ABBREVIATIONS THAT BEGIN WITH S

. . . .

Abbreviation	Meaning
r	right
RBC	red blood cell
re:	regarding
reg	regular
rehab	rehabilitation
resp	respirations
RLQ	right lower quadrant
RN	registered nurse
r/o	rule out
ROM	range of motion
rt	right
RUQ	right upper quadrant
Rx	treatment

Abbreviation	Meaning
sm	small
SOB	short of breath
s/p	status post
spec	specimen
SSE	soapsuds enema
ST	speech therapy
staph	staphylococcus
stat	immediately (*statin*)
STD	sexually transmitted disease
STI	sexually transmitted infection
strep	streptococcus
surg	surgery
Sx	symptom

Nursing Assistant/Nurse Aide Flash Review

ABBREVIATIONS THAT BEGIN WITH T

. . . .

ABBREVIATIONS THAT BEGIN WITH U, V, W & Y

. . . .

Abbreviation	Meaning
T	temperature
TB	tuberculosis
tbsp	tablespoon
TIA	transient ischemic attack
tid	three times a day (*ter in die*)
TPR	temperature, pulse, respiration
tsp	teaspoon
Tx	treatment or traction

Abbreviation	Meaning
U/A	urinalysis
URI	upper respiratory infection
UTI	urinary tract infection
VS	vital signs
WBC	white blood cell
w/c	wheelchair
WNL	within normal limits
w/o	without
wt or wgt	weight
w/u	workup
y/o	years old
yr	year

Nursing Assistant/Nurse Aide Flash Review

Body Systems

STRUCTURE OF THE INTEGUMENTARY SYSTEM

. . . .

FUNCTIONS OF THE INTEGUMENTARY SYSTEM

. . . .

The skin is made up of two layers:

1. The dermis is the deepest layer and consists of connective tissue. The dermis contains keratin, which helps skin cells thicken and become water resistant, and melanin, which is a brown or black pigment in the skin (e.g., freckles).

2. The epidermis is the outer layer of skin.

Sebaceous glands secrete an oily substance called sebum to keep the skin from drying out.

Sweat glands exist in two types:

1. Apocrine glands are found chiefly in the axilla and perineal area, become active when a person reaches puberty, and excrete a thick substance that creates body odor when it mixes with bacteria.

2. Eccrine glands cover most of the body and help cool the body through evaporation.

Hair is found over the entire body, except for the palms and soles. It develops from follicles in the dermis.

Nails are made up a skin cells that have been hardened by keratin.

· ·

The integumentary system provides the following functions:

- protection against harmful substances
- maintenance of fluid balance
- regulation of body temperature
- tactile sensation
- production of vitamin D
- absorption and elimination
- showing signs of the person's overall health (color, rashes)
- showing aspects of the person's personality (hair style, tattoos)

· ·

DIAGNOSTIC TESTS FOR INTEGUMENTARY SYSTEM DISORDERS

. . . .

BURNS

. . . .

CYANOSIS

Diagnostic tests for integumentary system disorders include:

- Tissue scrapings or biopsies are taken to identify lesions and other skin disorders.

- Skin tests are performed to check for allergies.

- Wood's lamp examination is used to detect fluorescent characteristics of certain skin infections.

. . . .

Burns are injuries to the skin and other tissue caused by heat or fire (thermal burns), electricity (electrical burns), chemicals (chemical burns), radiation (radiation burns, such as sunburn), or friction (friction burns). Burns are classified by their depth:

- Superficial (first degree): outer layer is damaged; painful and red.

- Partial thickness (second degree): epidermis and upper layer of dermis are damaged; red, blisters, painful, minimal scarring.

- Full thickness (third degree): epidermis and dermis are damaged; may involve underlying tissue; nerve endings are usually destroyed; skin is dark red to black to white, but usually there is no pain.

. . . .

Cyanosis is the blue or gray discoloration of the lips, nail beds, and skin caused by a lack of adequate oxygen. It is usually a sign of a respiratory or cardiac disorder.

EFFECTS OF AGING ON THE INTEGUMENTARY SYSTEM

PART 2

. . . .

ERYTHEMA (FLUSHING)

. . . .

INADEQUATE INTEGUMENTARY FUNCTION

The effects of aging on the integumentary system include:

- thin, fragile skin from loss of collagen
- slow healing from bruises due to decreased blood flow
- dry skin from decreased sebaceous glands
- age spots from increased melanin in the affected areas
- wrinkles from the loss of collagen
- graying of the hair due to loss of pigmentation
- thickening and yellowing of the nails due to decreased blood flow
- decreased ability to adjust to changes in temperature in the environment

Nursing assistants need to be aware that it is very easy to damage an elder's skin, and that elders may have more difficulty adjusting to heat and cold.

. . . .

Erythema is redness of the skin caused by increased blood flow in the capillaries and usually due to inflammation, infection, or injury.

. . . .

It is important that the nursing assistant observe for signs that a client is experiencing difficulty with the integumentary system. The nursing assistant should immediately report the following to the nurse when a client experiences:

- fever
- increased discomfort or pain
- new or increased redness, swelling, or warmth at a wound site
- change in wound drainage
- soaked or soiled dressing
- disconnected or pulled-out drainage tube
- malfunctioning vacuum-assisted closure (VAC) system

Nursing Assistant/Nurse Aide Flash Review

JAUNDICE

. . . .

MACULES AND PATCHES

. . . .

PALLOR

. . . .

PAPULES

Jaundice is yellow discoloration of the eyes and skin that is usually caused by a liver disorder.

. . . .

Macules are small, round, discolored flat spots that are less than one-half inch in diameter. A patch is a large macule. A freckle is a macule.

. . . .

Pallor is paleness. Some people have a normal pale coloring; however, pallor can also be caused by health problems such as anemia, illness, and shock.

. . . .

Papules are solid, raised lesions that are less than one-half inch in diameter. Causes of papules include psoriasis and skin cancer.

PRESSURE ULCER (DECUBITUS ULCER)

Bed sores are ulcers that develop when a body surface presses against a surface such as a mattress or bedpan for a long period of time. Risk factors include older age, poor nutrition, dehydration, cardiovascular or respiratory problems, moisture, friction (rubbing), and shearing (pulling). Pressure sores may be in one of four stages:

- Stage I: Skin is intact with signs of impending ulceration. The skin is red and warm to the touch. If the skin turns white, the blood flow has been compromised. Discoloration remains for more than 30 minutes after pressure is relieved.

- Stage II: There is a partial-thickness loss of skin that involves the epidermis and possibly dermis. It may appear as an abrasion, blister, or superficial ulceration.

- Stage III: There is a full-thickness loss of skin that extends into the sub-cutaneous tissue but not through the underlying fat. It may appear as a crater with or without drainage.

- Stage IV: There is full-thickness loss of skin and subcutaneous tissue that extends into muscle, bone, tendon, or joint capsule.

To prevent pressure sores, nursing assistants should:

- Avoid leaving clients in one position for a long period of time (no more than two hours).

- Promote good hydration and nutrition.

- Foster mobility.

- Provide good skin and perineal care.

- Assure that client toileting needs are met.

- Carefully monitor clients' skin.

- Make sure clothing is not too tight or too loose.

- Keep linens clean, dry. and wrinkle-free.

- Be gentle; use proper techniques to minimize rubbing and pulling of the skin.

- Use pressure-reducing devices, such as air or gel pads, elbow pads, and booties.

- Avoid massaging over bony areas.

When caring for a client with a pressure ulcer, the nursing assistant should inform the nurse of any of the following:

- redness over a pressure point that does not disappear after five minutes

- pain in an area over a pressure point

- a previously red area that becomes pale, white, or shiny

- change in the size or appearance of a pressure point

Nursing Assistant/Nurse Aide Flash Review

PUSTULE

. . . .

SHINGLES

. . . .

VACUUM-ASSISTED CLOSURE (VAC) THERAPY

PART
2

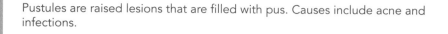

Pustules are raised lesions that are filled with pus. Causes include acne and infections.

. . . .

Shingles, also called herpes zoster, is a painful skin rash that is caused by the varicella zoster virus. It usually appears in a line or a small area on one side of the face or body. The condition occurs when the virus that causes chickenpox starts up again in a person's body.

. . . .

Vacuum-assisted closure (VAC) therapy is used for chronic or complicated wounds to promote healing. The VAC system applies negative pressure to the wound bed via a foam dressing. The foam fills the wound and is then connected via a suction tube to a canister that fits on the side of the vacuum pump unit. The system helps the wound by removing drainage and stimulating blood flow and the growth of new tissue.

Nursing Assistant/Nurse Aide Flash Review

VESICLES AND BLISTERS

. . . .

WOUNDS

. . . .

PART 2

A vesicle is a raised lesion that is filled with a clear fluid. A vesicle is less than one-quarter inch in diameter. Lesions of this type that are larger than one-quarter inch are called blisters or bullae. Causes of vesicles include sunburn, infections, or insect bites.

. . . .

Wounds are disruptions in the skin that may be intentional from planned medical or surgical intervention or unintentional from trauma. Wounds may be closed (bruises, redness, swelling) or open (incisions, lacerations).

Wound closure varies:

- Healing by first intention
    - also known as primary wound healing or primary closure
    - best choice for clean, fresh wounds in well-vascularized areas
    - wound closed surgically by sutures or staples

- Healing by second intention
    - also called secondary wound healing or spontaneous healing
    - used for contaminated or infected wounds and for pressure ulcers
    - wound left open to heal without surgical intervention

- Healing by third intention
    - also called tertiary wound healing or delayed primary closure
    - useful for wounds that are too contaminated for primary closure but appear clean and well vascularized
    - wound left open for a period of time, then surgically repaired with sutures or staples

Wounds may also be treated with drains to remove collected fluids or with dressings to absorb excessive drainage or promote a moist environment, protect the wound bed, and decrease the risk of infection. Montgomery ties or straps may be used in place of tape for large wounds, especially surgical wounds of the abdomen. Chronic or complicated wounds may require vacuum-assisted closure (VAC) therapy to promote healing.

. . . .

Nursing Assistant/Nurse Aide Flash Review

PART 2

STRUCTURE OF THE RESPIRATORY SYSTEM

. . . .

FUNCTIONS OF THE RESPIRATORY SYSTEM

. . . .

DIAGNOSTIC TESTS FOR RESPIRATORY SYSTEM DISORDERS

The respiratory system includes the following components:

- The nasal cavity conditions the air that is received by the nose by warming or cooling the air, removing dust particles from it, and moistening it before it enters the pharynx.

- The pharynx is behind the nasal cavity and above the larynx, and it also serves as part of the digestive system because food as well as air passes through the pharynx.

- The larynx produces sound when air causes the vocal cords to vibrate. The larynx is in the neck and plays a vital role in the protection of the trachea.

- The trachea is located in the neck and chest and is made up of cartilage to keep it open.

- The bronchi branch off the trachea, and further divide into bronchiole tubes.

- The lungs are the most important component of the respiratory system, as they are responsible for transporting oxygen from the atmosphere into blood and releasing carbon dioxide from blood to the atmosphere.

. . . .

The functions of the respiratory system are:

- ventilation or breathing—the movement of air in and out of the lungs

- gas exchange—transporting oxygen to the blood and releasing carbon dioxide into the atmosphere

. . . .

Diagnostic tests for respiratory system disorders include:

- Chest X-rays are performed to create pictures of the heart and lungs and assist in finding the causes of symptoms such as coughing.

- Pulmonary function tests measure how well the lungs take in and release air, as well as how they move gases such as oxygen from the atmosphere into the body's circulation.

- Blood gases determine if the lungs are functioning well enough to exchange oxygen and carbon dioxide.

- Pulse oximetry monitors the client's saturation of oxygen in his or her blood.

ASTHMA

. . . .

BRONCHITIS

. . . .

CHRONIC OBSTRUCTIVE PULMONARY DISEASE (COPD)

Asthma affects the bronchi and bronchioles and can be caused by allergies. Asthmatic triggers such as cigarette smoke, cold weather, allergens, exercise, and infections cause the bronchi and bronchioles to narrow to the point where breathing becomes difficult, often causing the client to wheeze.

. . . .

Bronchitis is an inflammation of the bronchi that is usually caused by an infection and that can turn into pneumonia if not treated.

. . . .

COPD is a term used to describe emphysema and chronic bronchitis. Both of these disorders can exist in the same person, and both are often caused by smoking.

- Emphysema involves damage to the alveoli. Therefore the client no longer has effective gas (oxygen and carbon dioxide) exchange. Air gets trapped in the enlarged alveoli, as does fluid, which creates a suitable environment for infectious organisms to grow. Clients with emphysema have difficulty breathing. Their breathing is shallow and rapid, and they may have to catch their breath when engaging in physical activity or even talking. Clients with emphysema may also have enlarged chests (barrel chests) due to years of air being trapped in their lungs.

- Chronic bronchitis results from chronic irritation to the bronchi and bronchioles. The irritation causes the production of thick mucus that blocks airways, interferes with breathing, and creates a breeding ground for infectious organisms. Clients with chronic bronchitis have chest tightness, difficulty breathing, and a chronic productive cough.

Nursing Assistant/Nurse Aide Flash Review

EFFECTS OF AGING ON THE RESPIRATORY SYSTEM

. . . .

INADEQUATE OXYGENATION

. . . .

LUNG CANCER

The effects of aging on the respiratory system include:

- The respiratory system's effectiveness can be decreased by immobility, chronic illness, and long-term exposure to toxins such as tobacco smoke, coal dust, and asbestos.
- Loss of tissue elasticity and decreased muscle tone can result in ineffective ventilation.
- Decreased immune function can result in increased risk for respiratory infection.

• •

It is important that the nursing assistant observe for signs that a client is experiencing difficulty with ventilation or gas exchange. Nursing assistants should know their clients' normal color and should immediately report to the nurse when a client experiences any of the following:

- sudden chest pain or difficulty breathing
- very slow or shallow respirations
- ceased respirations
- shortness of breath during activity that the client tolerated before
- blue or gray coloring in the lips, nail beds, or skin (referred to as cyanosis)
- noising breathing (wheezing, gurgling sounds, crowing, barking)
- coughing up discolored sputum (yellow, green, brown, red-streaked, frothy)
- improper oxygen flow rate on meter
- pulse oximetry reading below 92%
- low reading on gauge on oxygen tank
- dislodged tracheostomy or endotracheal tube

• •

Lung cancer is one of the most common causes of cancer-related deaths in the United States, and people who smoke are ten times more likely to develop lung cancer than those who do not.

MECHANICAL VENTILATION

....

OXYGEN THERAPY

....

PNEUMONIA

Mechanical ventilation is used for clients who cannot breathe on their own. These clients are intubated with a tracheostomy or an endotracheal tube.

. . . .

Room air contains approximately 20% oxygen, and clients with poor lung function may not be able to get the oxygen they need from breathing room air. Therefore, their physicians may prescribe oxygen therapy with 100% oxygen, which can be given as needed or continuously. Oxygen may be delivered through a wall-mounted system, a pressurized tank, or an oxygen concentrator and supplied from a nasal cannula or face mask. When working with oxygen, the nursing assistant should:

- Make sure the equipment is in working order (e.g., no frayed cords).
- Avoid any type of flame in the person's room (e.g., lighted match, cigarette, candle).
- Keep oxygen tubing kink free.
- Know the client's flow rate, but avoid adjusting the flow rate.
- Avoid removing the nasal cannula or mask unless instructed to do so by the nurse.
- Make sure the humidity bottle water level is not too low.
- Provide oral care as directed by the nurse.
- Monitor the skin near the tubing for signs of irritation.

. . . .

Pneumonia is an inflammation of the lungs that may be caused by infection. The alveoli fill with fluid and pus, which prevents air from entering them, resulting in decrease gas exchange (oxygen cannot get in, and carbon dioxide cannot get out). Aspiration pneumonia occurs when foreign material (vomit, saliva, food, beverages) is inhaled into the lungs. Unconscious clients and clients receiving tube feedings are at increased risk for aspiration pneumonia because they cannot protect their airways.

SUCTIONING

. . . .

TRACHEOSTOMY

. . . .

Suctioning is used to clear the airway of secretions. A suction tube is connected to a vacuum device and canister. The tip of the tube is placed into the person's nose or mouth, and the vacuum starts to remove the secretions. Suctioning is also used for endotracheal and tracheostomy tubes. Since suctioning also removes air, the client can become hypoxic (oxygen deficient). Nursing assistants typically do not suction clients; however, they are responsible for notifying the nurse when a client needs suctioning.

· ·

A tracheostomy (or trach) is a surgically created opening in the trachea that may be temporary or permanent. It is performed as an emergency procedure when the upper airway is obstructed, when the larynx is removed because of cancer, or when a person is placed on mechanical ventilation. A tracheostomy tube is inserted into the opening and secured around the person's neck. The person breathes through the tracheostomy instead of the mouth, but can still drink and eat.

· ·

Nursing Assistant/Nurse Aide Flash Review

STRUCTURE OF THE CARDIOVASCULAR SYSTEM

PART 2

. . . .

FUNCTIONS OF THE CARDIOVASCULAR SYSTEM

. . . .

DIAGNOSTIC TESTS FOR CARDIOVASCULAR SYSTEM DISORDERS

The heart is a muscle that is made up of two sides and four chambers: the left and right atria and the left and right ventricles. The atria are located on the top of the heart and receive blood from the body, while the ventricles are located on the bottom of the heart and pump blood away to the body. The right ventricle pumps deoxygenated blood to the lungs. The left ventricle pumps oxygenated blood to the rest of the body. There are valves between the chambers, and these control the flow of blood, making sure that it flows in one direction. The four valves are the tricuspid valve, the pulmonic or pulmonary valve, the mitral valve, and the aortic valve.

The blood vessels are tubes that carry blood to and from the heart. They include arteries (carry oxygenated blood to the body, except for the pulmonary artery), veins (carry deoxygenated blood back to the heart, (except for the pulmonary vein), and capillaries that enable the nutrients to get to the cells and carbon dioxide to get back into the bloodstream for removal.

• •

The functions of the cardiovascular system are:

• transporting oxygen and nutrients to the body

• temperature regulation

• •

Diagnostic tests for cardiovascular system disorders include:

• Doppler ultrasound is used to check the blood flow of large arteries and veins.

• Chest X-ray shows the size of the heart and checks for enlargement.

• Electrocardiogram (ECG, EKG) shows abnormalities in the heart's conduction system.

• Stress test is an ECG while exercising.

• Echocardiogram uses sound waves to assess various heart problems.

ANGINA PECTORIS

. . . .

ANTICOAGULANT MEDICATION

. . . .

ATHEROSCLEROSIS

PART 2

Angina pectoris is the chest pain felt when the heart muscle is deprived of oxygen. The pain may be felt in the middle of the chest, or it may start in the chest and go to the arm or neck—clients experience it differently. Clients may also feel very anxious or like they are suffocating. Clients with chronic angina use nitroglycerin pills to relieve the pain. These pills work by relaxing the arteries and increasing blood flow. Nursing assistants who are trained to help administer nitroglycerin to clients need to avoid handling these pills with their bare hands because the medication can absorb through the skin and cause a drop in blood pressure and a bad headache.

· ·

Anticoagulant medications or blood thinners are used to prevent clots from forming. Clients taking these medications are at risk for bleeding. The nursing assistants should immediately report:

- any signs of bleeding or bruising in the skin

- bleeding from any area of the body (mouth, nose, anus)

- blood in the urine or stool

· ·

Atherosclerosis is blockage of the arteries by fatty plaques. This causes less oxygen and nutrition to get to the body cells. Plaque can also cause blood clots to form. These can break off and become emboli, which can travel to arteries in major organs and cause serious and sometimes fatal consequences, including stroke, heart attack, and kidney failure.

Nursing Assistant/Nurse Aide Flash Review

CORONARY ARTERY DISEASE (CAD)

. . . .

DYSRHYTHMIA

. . . .

EDEMA

Coronary artery disease (CAD) is the leading cause of death in the United States. CAD results from narrowing of the coronary arteries due to atherosclerosis. The coronary arteries supply blood to the heart; thus the heart muscle may not receive adequate oxygen and nutrition during activity. Over time, the arteries may become so narrow that no blood gets through and parts of the heart muscle die. CAD may be treated with medications, balloon angioplasty, or a surgery called coronary artery bypass graft (CABG). A stent (mesh tube) may be placed during the angioplasty to provide support for the artery wall.

. . . .

A dysrhythmia, also called arrhythmia, is an irregular heart rate and/or rhythm that can cause clients to experience fatigue, dizziness, fainting, and heart palpitations. They can also increase a client's risk of heart attack or stroke. Dysrhythmias can be caused by coronary artery disease, electrolyte imbalance, changes in the heart muscle, heart attack, or heart surgery. There are also many types of dysrhythmias, including atrial fibrillation and premature ventricular contractions (PVCs). They can be treated with medications to control the heart rate and anticoagulants to prevent stroke. Other treatments include cardioversion, pacemaker placement, and cardiac ablation (destruction of a function).

. . . .

Edema is abnormal swelling due to the buildup of fluid. It is most commonly seen in the ankles, legs, hands, and abdomen.

EFFECTS OF AGING ON THE CARDIOVASCULAR SYSTEM

. . . .

EMBOLISM

. . . .

HEART FAILURE

The effects of aging on the cardiovascular system include:

- less efficient contraction of the heart
- possible enlarged heart from overworking
- loss of elasticity in the arteries and veins
- buildup of fatty deposits (atherosclerosis) in blood vessels

. . . .

An embolus is usually a part of a thrombus that breaks free and travels though the bloodstream until it gets stuck in a narrow artery and causes a blockage. Emboli can also be caused by pieces of plaque, fat, air, or other substances. A cerebral embolus is an embolus in the brain (causes a stroke); a pulmonary embolus is an embolus in the lung. Both are medical emergencies; therefore, the nurse should be alerted.

. . . .

The heart fails when it is unable to pump enough blood for the body's needs. This does not mean that it has stopped. Right-sided heart failure is also called *cor pulmonale*, and left-sided heart failure is called *congestive heart failure*. Causes of heart failure include coronary artery disease, myocardial infarction, heart valve disease, infections, drug or alcohol abuse, heart defects, diabetes, and kidney disease. Symptoms include fatigue and weakness; dizziness; shortness of breath; dry, hacky cough; fluid retention (edema); and rapid or irregular heartbeats. Heart failure is treated with medications and usually a cardiac or low-sodium diet. Many times oxygen treatment is also required.

Nursing Assistant/Nurse Aide Flash Review

INADEQUATE CARDIOVASCULAR FUNCTIONING

. . . .

MYOCARDIAL INFARCTION (MI)

. . . .

It is important that the nursing assistant observe for signs that a client is experiencing a cardiovascular problem. The nursing assistant should report the following to the nurse immediately:

- chest pain, pressure, squeezing, or burning
- pain in the shoulder, arm, neck, throat, jaw, or back
- palpitations
- nausea
- weakness, fatigue, or dizziness
- sweating
- cyanosis of the lips, nail beds, and/or skin
- slow or rapid irregular pulse
- unusually high or low blood pressure
- difficulty breathing
- decreased tolerance for usual physical activities
- blue or gray discoloration of the legs or feet
- decreased pulses in the lower extremities
- coldness in the lower extremities
- painful swelling of the legs, especially the calves
- painful, swollen red areas on the extremities, especially the legs

• •

Myocardial infarction (MI) is also called a heart attack. One or more of the coronary arteries blocks completely. This prevents blood from reaching parts of the heart muscle and oxygenating them. The muscle areas then die (infarct). Severity depends on the location and the extent of the damage. Atrial MIs may not be life-threatening; however, ventricular MIs can be fatal because they reduce the heart's ability to pump blood to vital organs. Early detection and treatment increase a person's chances of survival.

• •

Nursing Assistant/Nurse Aide Flash Review

PACEMAKER

· ·

PHLEBITIS

· ·

RISK FACTORS FOR HEART DISEASE

PART
2

A pacemaker is a battery-operated device that is surgically implanted under the skin in the chest. It looks and feels like a small square or circular box. It sends electrical impulses to the heart muscle to keep an adequate heart rate.

· ·

Phlebitis occurs when blood pools in the veins and causes the lining of the veins to become inflamed. The affected area is usually painful, red, hard, and hot to the touch. When caused by a clot, this is called thrombophlebitis, and when in the deep veins it is called deep vein thrombophlebitis (DVT). In the latter, a clot can break off and travel to the lung, causing a pulmonary embolism, which is potentially life-threatening. DVT can be caused by prolonged sitting in a car or plane and becoming dehydrated, and by prolonged bed rest, surgery, obesity, cancer, and trauma to the lower body. Older people are also more at risk for DVT.

· ·

Risk factors for heart disease are:

- Nonmodifiable (cannot change) risk factors:
  - increased age
  - male gender (females are equally at risk after menopause)
  - family history of heart disease
  - body shape: increased weight around the chest and abdomen (apple shape)

- Modifiable (can change) risk factors:
  - smoking
  - physical inactivity
  - obesity or overweight
  - excessive alcohol use
  - diet high in saturated fat, sodium, and cholesterol
  - poorly controlled high blood pressure
  - poorly controlled diabetes
  - high cholesterol

THROMBUS

. . . .

VARICOSE VEINS

. . . .

VENOUS STASIS ULCERS

A thrombus is a blood clot that forms locally in a vessel (also see embolism). Prevention in the hospital usually involves the use of sequential compression devices (SCDs) on the lower legs. Note: Never massage legs, as doing so would increase the risk of a potential or actual thrombus becoming an embolus.

. . . .

Varicose veins are large, swollen, twisted blood vessels that usually develop in the legs. Clients with varicose veins experience pain and cramping in their legs, and sometimes heaviness, throbbing, and tingling. Risk factors include occupations that involve frequent standing (nurses, nursing assistants, hairdressers), as well as heredity, obesity, pregnancy, and birth control pills. Treatment includes wearing support stockings; lifestyle changes (proper skin hygiene, weight loss); sclerotherapy (injections into veins); and laser treatment. Varicose veins can place the client at risk for phlebitis or stasis ulcers.

. . . .

Venous stasis ulcers tend to occur near the ankles and result when the pressure of pooled blood in the veins forces plasma out of the veins and into the tissues. The area becomes inflamed, swollen, and fragile, eventually breaking down into an open sore. Symptoms include pain and mobility difficulty. Prevention and treatment include the use of antiembolism stockings and leg exercises.

PART
2

STRUCTURE OF THE DIGESTIVE SYSTEM

. . . .

The digestive system includes the following components:

- The mouth is the beginning of the digestive tract. Digestion begins when food is chewed and mixed with saliva.

- The esophagus receives food from the mouth after swallowing and delivers it to the stomach.

- The stomach holds food as it is being mixed with enzymes that continue the process of breaking down food into a usable form for digestion to continue.

- The small intestine is a 22-foot-long tube that is made up of the duodenum, jejunum, and ileum. It breaks down food using enzymes from the pancreas and bile from the liver. Peristalsis moves food through, mixing it with the digestive secretions from the pancreas and liver. Contents start out in a semisolid form and end in a liquid form after passing through the entire small intestine.

- The pancreas secretes digestive enzymes into the small intestine to break down protein, fats, and carbohydrates. The pancreas also makes insulin, the chief hormone for metabolizing sugar.

- The liver has multiple functions. Its main function within the digestive system is to process the nutrients absorbed from the small intestine.

- The gallbladder stores bile and releases it into the duodenum to help absorb and digest fats.

- The colon or large intestine connects the small intestine to the rectum and is made up of the cecum, the ascending (right) colon, the transverse (across) colon, the descending (left) colon, and the sigmoid colon. The appendix is attached to the cecum. The colon processes waste so that emptying the bowels is easy and convenient.

- The rectum connects the colon to the anus. It receives stool from the colon and holds it until evacuation happens.

- The anus is surrounded by sphincter muscles that are important in allowing control of stool. The external sphincter holds the stool until reaching a toilet, where it then relaxes to release the contents.

Nursing Assistant/Nurse Aide Flash Review

FUNCTIONS OF THE DIGESTIVE SYSTEM

· ·

DIAGNOSTIC TESTS FOR DIGESTIVE SYSTEM DISORDERS

· ·

CANCER

The functions of the digestive system are:

- ingestion: taking food and fluids into the body
- digestion: breaking down food into simple elements for absorption
- absorption: absorbing nutrients from food
- elimination: excreting bodily wastes

. . . .

Diagnostic tests for digestive system disorders include:

- Upper endoscopy is used to look inside the esophagus, stomach, and duodenum to discover the reason for swallowing difficulties, nausea, vomiting, reflux, bleeding, indigestion, abdominal pain, or chest pain.
- The upper gastrointestinal series uses X-rays to diagnose problems in the esophagus, stomach, and duodenum, and possibly the rest of the small intestine.
- The lower gastrointestinal series uses X-rays to diagnose problems in the colon and rectum. It may show problems like abnormal growths, ulcers, polyps, and diverticuli.
- Colonoscopy allows the physician to look inside the entire large intestine, and is used to look for cancer and other colon problems.
- Sigmoidoscopy allows the physician to look inside the sigmoid colon. This may be used to find the cause of diarrhea, abdominal pain, or constipation or to look for cancer.

. . . .

Cancer can strike any part of the digestive tract. Symptoms depend on severity and location, but may include loss of appetite, pain, indigestion, vomiting, changes in stool patterns, and blood in the stool.

CONSTIPATION

. . . .

DIARRHEA

. . . .

EFFECTS OF AGING ON THE DIGESTIVE SYSTEM

Normal aging increases the risk for constipation, as do poor diet, decreased fluid intake, some medications, and poor bowel habits. Constipation may be treated with bowel training, dietary fiber intake, increased fluid intake, exercise, and laxatives.

. . . .

Diarrhea can be acute or chronic and can result in dehydration, and thus should be reported to the nurse. There are many causes of diarrhea. Common causes in older adults include medication, diverticulitis, diabetes, and infections. Older people are more susceptible to nosocomial (hospital-based) diarrhea, especially after taking antibiotics for other infections.

. . . .

The effects of aging on the digestive system include:

- Many older people have missing teeth or dentures, which can interfere with chewing and swallowing, creating choking hazards.

- Saliva production decreases. This can make chewing and swallowing more difficult.

- Loss of muscle tone can cause incontinence and constipation.

- Production of digestive enzymes slows, making digestion more difficult.

- Constipation is not a physiologic effect of old age; however, movement through the digestive tract slows, which may result in constipation. Some medications may also increase this risk.

GALLBLADDER DISORDERS

. . . .

HERNIAS

. . . .

ULCERS

PART 2

Gallbladder disease usually results from the buildup of stones in the gallbladder, which block the flow of bile into the duodenum. This causes episodic severe pain in the right upper abdomen that may spread to the right shoulder and back. Since bile is needed to digest fat, people with gallbladder disease may have pale, clay-colored stools that float because of their fat content. Gallstones may be treated with medications or laser treatment or surgical removal of the gallbladder.

. . . .

Hernias occur when fatty tissue or organs protrude through a weak spot in abdominal muscle or connective tissue. They can also occur in an old abdominal surgical incision. Common hernias are:

- femoral: outer groin
- hiatal: upper stomach
- inguinal: inner groin
- umbilical: naval

If the muscles tighten around the protruding tissue and cut off the blood supply, the result is a strangulated hernia. This is a surgical emergency. Signs of a strangulated hernia are pain, nausea, vomiting, and fever. If anyone with a hernia has a sudden onset or increase in pain, inform the nurse immediately.

. . . .

Ulcers are erosions in skin or mucosa. In the digestive tract, the common ulcers are found in the stomach (gastric ulcer) and the duodenum (duodenal ulcer). Clients with ulcers may feel nauseated or uncomfortably full after eating. However, if the ulcer eats through the stomach lining and perforates, the client will probably experience severe pain, nausea, and vomiting. If these symptoms occur, inform the nurse immediately.

Nursing Assistant/Nurse Aide Flash Review

PART 2

STRUCTURE OF THE URINARY SYSTEM

....

FUNCTIONS OF THE URINARY SYSTEM

....

DIAGNOSTIC TESTS FOR URINARY SYSTEM DISORDERS

The urinary system includes the following components:

- The kidneys contain nephrons that filter urea from blood. Nephrons are filtering units that consist of a blood vessel called a capillary and a urine-collecting tube called the renal tubule. The kidneys also release critical hormones for red blood cell production, blood pressure regulation, and calcium regulation.

- The bladder stores urine until the body is ready to excrete it.

- The ureters are small tubes that connect the kidneys and bladder and carry urine.

- The urethra is the tube that brings urine from the bladder to outside the body.

· ·

The functions of the urinary system are:

- removing liquid wastes

- maintaining homeostasis (fluids, electrolytes, and acid/base balance)

· ·

Diagnostic tests for urinary system disorders include:

- The urinalysis examines the physical, chemical, and microscopic makeup of urine.

- The urine culture is a clean catch urine sample that is used to test for bacteria, and to detect the cause of a urinary tract infection.

- A 24-hour urine test checks for the presence of proteins to diagnose conditions that affect kidney function, such as nephrotic syndrome and glomerulonephritis.

- A urine pregnancy test detects the presence of the hormone known as human chorionic gonadotropin (HCG), which is in the urine of pregnant women in the first trimester. Cystoscopy is an examination of the bladder using a scope.

- Ultrasound may be used to detect tumors and abnormalities in the urinary tract.

Nursing Assistant/Nurse Aide Flash Review

CANCER

. . . .

EFFECTS OF AGING ON THE URINARY SYSTEM

. . . .

INADEQUATE URINARY FUNCTIONING

PART 2

Cancer of the bladder is common among smokers, and risk increases with age. If treatment requires removal of the bladder and the creation of a urinary diversion, such as a ureterostomy (ureters drain into an ostomy appliance) or a urostomy (ureters are attached to a section of the small intestine, usually the ileum [illeal conduit], and the section of intestine is sealed off and brought through the abdominal wall where a stoma is created). These procedures may also be used for people with spinal cord injuries or spina bifida (birth defect). Clients with urinary diversions require good skin care and observation for skin and urinary infections.

. . . .

The effects of aging on the urinary system include:

- loss of muscle tone, leading to reduced bladder capacity, greater frequency (need to urinate at frequent intervals), nocturia (abnormal need to urinate through nighttime hours), and stress incontinence

- decreased ability to filter waste

- increased risk for urinary infections because of incomplete emptying of the bladder

- prostate enlargement in males, which can result in urinary dribbling and slow start of urinary stream when voiding

. . . .

It is important that the nursing assistant observe for signs that a client is experiencing a urinary problem. These signs should be reported to the nurse immediately:

- change in alertness and/or orientation, or unusual behavior

- a major increase or decrease in the volume of urine over a period of time

- blood in the urine

- sudden, sharp pain in the abdomen, back, or side

- burning or pain on urination

- change in voiding patterns

- urine that is foul smelling, is cloudy, or has an unusual color

Nursing Assistant/Nurse Aide Flash Review

PART 2

KIDNEY FAILURE

. . . .

Kidney (renal) failure is the loss of the kidneys' ability to filter waste and excess fluids from the body. Wastes and fluids build up, causing the person to become very ill. Kidney failure can be acute or chronic.

- Acute kidney failure develops quickly over a few hours to a few days and is common in people who are already hospitalized. It can have many causes, but they generally can be categorized under conditions that slow blood flow to the kidneys (e.g., heart failure, infection, severe allergic reaction, severe burns); directly damage the kidneys (e.g., blood clots, medications, glomerulonephritis, toxins); or cause blockage to the urinary drainage tubes (e.g., cancer, enlarged prostate, kidney stones). Symptoms include decreased urinary output, fluid retention, drowsiness, confusion, chest pain, and seizures. Acute kidney failure can be fatal; it requires rapid treatment, but may be reversible.

- Chronic failure is a gradual loss of kidney function. It may be caused by illnesses, such as diabetes, hypertension, and kidney infections. Symptoms appear slowly over time, and include hypertension, fatigue, nausea and vomiting, muscle twitches and cramps, persistent itching, and changes in urine output).

People in renal failure are often treated with dialysis. In hemodialysis, the person's blood is passed intravenously through a machine that filters the body waste. The person has a fistula or graft created prior to dialysis to create a long-term access point for needles and tubing. In peritoneal dialysis, solutions that absorb waste are added to the person's abdominal cavity and later drained after they absorb waste. Persons with chronic kidney failure need to remain on dialysis for life, unless they receive a kidney transplant. Care of a client in renal failure includes:

- vital signs while avoiding taking blood pressure readings in the arm with a fistula
- accurate intake and output
- assistance with activities of daily living
- frequent repositioning and range of motion exercises
- frequent skin care
- collection of urine samples as directed

KIDNEY STONES

....

NEUROGENIC BLADDER

....

URINARY TRACT INFECTIONS

Kidney stones, also called renal calculi, develop when mineral salt wastes concentrate and form crystals that continue to grow in size. Risk factors include not drinking enough, immobility, and urinary infections; however, kidney stones can also be caused by neurogenic bladder, prostate enlargement, and a weakened bladder wall. Symptoms include pain and blood in the urine. When caring for clients with kidney stones, nursing assistants are often instructed to collect and strain the client's urine to retrieve the stones so that they can be sent to the laboratory for chemical analysis.

· ·

Neurogenic bladder is a lack of bladder control due to a brain, spinal cord, or nerve condition, including spina bifida, cerebral palsy, encephalitis, multiple sclerosis, spinal cord injury, and brain or spinal cord tumors. There are two types of neurogenic bladder:

1. Underactive: The bladder cannot contract. It is flaccid and becomes overstretched, resulting in increased bladder capacity. However, because of nerve damage, the person may not be able to tell the bladder is full, resulting in reflex incontinence as the bladder empties automatically. Treatment may include intermittent or continuous catheterization.

2. Overactive: The bladder is spastic and sensitive to stimulation. The muscles contract involuntarily, pushing urine out and causing incontinence.

Urinary incontinence can cause embarrassment for clients; therefore, the nursing assistant can help them with hygiene so that they feel fresh and clean.

· ·

Urinary tract infections can occur in the urethra, bladder, or kidneys, and can occur at any age. Symptoms of lower urinary tract infections include frequency, urgency, and burning. Kidney infections may have more serious symptoms and can cause permanent damage to the kidneys if not treated promptly.

STRUCTURE OF THE MALE REPRODUCTIVE SYSTEM

. . . .

STRUCTURE OF THE FEMALE REPRODUCTIVE SYSTEM

. . . .

The male reproductive system includes the following components:

- The penis is used in sexual intercourse. It contains the root (attaches to the wall of the abdomen), the shaft (body), and the glans (head). The head of the penis is covered with the foreskin, which may have been removed via a circumcision, and it contains the urethra that transports semen and urine. When a man is sexually aroused, the penis fills with blood and becomes rigid and erect, to allow for penetration during sexual intercourse.

- The scrotum is a pouchlike sac of skin that hangs behind and below the penis. It contains the testicles (testes), as well as many nerves and blood vessels.

- The testes make testosterone, the primary male sex hormone, and generate sperm in their seminiferous tubules.

· ·

The female reproductive system has both external and internal structures.

The external structures include:

- The labia majora covers the other external reproductive organs. They contain sweat and oil-secreting glands and are covered with hair after puberty.

- The labia minora lie just inside the labia majora, and surround the openings to the vagina.

- The clitoris is very sensitive to stimulation and can become erect.

The internal structures include:

- The vagina is known as the birth canal.

- The uterus is the home to a developing fetus. It contains the cervix, which is the lower part that opens into the vagina, and the body of the uterus, called the corpus. An opening in the cervix allows sperm to enter and menstrual blood to exit.

- The ovaries produce eggs and hormones.

- The fallopian tubes connect the uterus and ovaries. Conception normally occurs in the fallopian tubes.

The female reproductive system also includes the breasts (mammary glands), which are made up of ducts, fat, muscle, and glandular tissue.

· ·

Nursing Assistant/Nurse Aide Flash Review

FUNCTIONS OF THE MALE REPRODUCTIVE SYSTEM

. . . .

FUNCTIONS OF THE FEMALE REPRODUCTIVE SYSTEM

. . . .

DIAGNOSTIC TESTS FOR REPRODUCTIVE SYSTEM DISORDERS

PART 2

The functions of the male reproductive system are:

- to produce and transport sperm (the male reproductive cells) and protective fluid (semen)

- to eject sperm

- to produce and secrete male sex hormones to maintain the male reproductive system

. . . .

The functions of the female reproductive system are:

- preparation for pregnancy

- reproduction

- to produce and secrete female sex hormones to maintain the female reproductive system

- to produce and provide nourishment for an infant

. . . .

Diagnostic tests for reproductive system disorders include:

- Blood work may be collected to check hormone levels.

- Biopsies may be performed to check for cancer.

- Mammograms are used to screen for breast cancer.

AMENORRHEA

. . . .

CANCER—FEMALES

. . . .

CANCER—MALES

Amenorrhea is the absence of menstrual periods. Primary amenorrhea, which means a female has not menstruated by age 16, can be caused by poor nutrition, hormonal problems, or disorders of the reproductive organs. Secondary amenorrhea, which means a female loses her periods, can be caused by pregnancy, hormonal imbalances, stress, participation in extensive athletics, or tumors.

. . . .

- According to the Center for Disease Control and Prevention, breast cancer is the most common cancer in women in the United States. Breast self-exam (BSE) is no longer recommended as a screening tool for breast cancer; however, it can help women learn the normal feeling of their breasts and report changes in their breasts early on to their healthcare provider.

- Cervical cancer is most common between the ages of 30 and 50. Risk factors include human papilloma virus (HPV), having sexual intercourse at a young age, and having multiple sex partners.

- Endometrial cancer, which is also called uterine cancer, is more common after menopause.

- Ovarian cancer most commonly occurs between the ages of 40 and 65 and is the leading cause of cancer-related death in women.

. . . .

- Penile cancer is a less common cancer, but may be the cause of penile lesions; thus, such lesions should be reported.

- Prostate cancer is more commonly seen in men over age 50 and has a good cure rate if discovered and treated early.

- Testicular cancer usually affects young and middle-aged males and can spread quickly if not detected early. Testicular self-exam may help males detect lumps in their early stage.

CYSTOCELE

. . . .

EFFECTS OF AGING ON THE REPRODUCTIVE SYSTEM

. . . .

HYSTERECTOMY

A cystocele is the downward shifting of the bladder to where it presses on the anterior portion of the vagina. Cystoceles can cause stress incontinence and incomplete emptying of the bladder.

. . . .

The effects of aging on the male reproductive system include:

- Males remain fertile but there is decreased production of testosterone and sperm.
- Erections last for shorter periods of time and occur less frequently.
- The prostate enlarges and may make urination difficult.
- Medications, including those taken for high blood pressure, can affect sexual functioning.

The effects of aging on the female reproductive system include:

- Menopause occurs around age 45 to 55.
- Decreased hormone production may cause some women to develop facial hair and a deeper voice.
- The vagina becomes dry, which can make intercourse difficult without lubrication.

. . . .

A hysterectomy is the surgical removal of the uterus for cancer, excessive bleeding, or other problems. This can also cause stress because the woman can no longer bear children.

IMPOTENCE

· ·

INADEQUATE FEMALE REPRODUCTIVE FUNCTIONING

· ·

INADEQUATE MALE REPRODUCTIVE FUNCTIONING

Also called erectile dysfunction (ED), impotence is the inability to achieve an erection long enough to engage in sexual activity. It may be temporary or permanent and can be caused by low levels of male hormones, medications, circulation problems, or emotional issues. Impotence can cause emotional distress to the point that the affected male may not even want to report it to his healthcare provider.

. . . .

It is important that the nursing assistant observe for signs that a female client is experiencing a reproductive problem. The following signs should be reported to the nurse immediately:

- unusual discharge from the nipples
- lump or thickened area in the breast
- puckering in the skin of the breasts
- unusual vaginal discharge
- unusual vaginal bleeding, especially after menopause
- very heavy menstrual bleeding
- lower abdominal pain or cramping
- pelvic pressure or cramping
- difficulty emptying the bladder
- protrusion from the vagina
- itching or burning around the vagina
- inflammation of the vulva
- lesions or thickened areas in the genital area

. . . .

It is important that the nursing assistant observe for signs that a male client is experiencing a reproductive problem. The following signs should be reported to the nurse immediately:

- changes in the skin in the genital area
- unusual or bloody discharge from the penis
- pain or burning on urination
- pain in the scrotal or rectal area

INFERTILITY

....

MASTECTOMY

....

RECTOCELE

Infertility is the inability to become pregnant or cause a woman to become pregnant. It can be caused by the inability to produce adequate sperm in males, or problems with the female reproductive system.

· ·

A mastectomy is the surgical removal of the breast because of breast cancer that cannot be treated in another manner, such as a lumpectomy. This surgery can be emotionally difficult for women, and thus women who have this surgery need emotional support. There are also some women who choose this procedure when they are at high risk for breast cancer.

· ·

A rectocele is the downward shifting of the front wall of the rectum to where it presses into the posterior of the vaginal wall. Rectoceles can cause a feeling of pressure in the rectum and difficulty having a bowel movement.

SEXUALLY TRANSMITTED INFECTIONS (STIs)

. . . .

UTERINE PROLAPSE

. . . .

Once called venereal diseases and sexually transmitted diseases, STIs are transmitted through penile and vaginal secretions. They include HIV/AIDS, herpes, gonorrhea, chlamydia, genital warts, and syphilis. Some STIs may cause no symptoms, whereas HIV/AIDS can affect the entire body.

. . . .

Uterine prolapse is the downward shifting of the uterus into the vagina. It may even be visible outside the vagina. This can cause feelings of fullness and difficulty with urination and defecation.

. . . .

PART
2

STRUCTURE OF THE MUSCULOSKELETAL SYSTEM

. . . .

FUNCTIONS OF THE MUSCULOSKELETAL SYSTEM

. . . .

The skeletal system consists of 206 bones that include long, short, flat, and irregular bones.

Joints are the junctions between two or more bones. Ligaments connect bone to bone to form joints.

- Fixed joints do not move (joints between bones of the skull).
- Hinge joints allow only bending (joints in the knees, fingers, and toes).
- Ball-and-socket joints allow inward and outward rotation, as well as forward, backward, and sideways movement (joints in the shoulders and hips).

There are three types of muscle:

1. Skeletal muscle contracts to move body parts.
2. Cardiac muscle forms the heart, but is not part of the musculoskeletal system.
3. Smooth muscle covers many arteries and contracts to help blood flow; it also works in the digestive tract.

Tendons are bands of connective tissue that attach each end of a muscle to a bone.

Cartilage is found at the end of bones (e.g., the nose).

· ·

The functions of the musculoskeletal system are:

- giving shape to the body
- protecting vital organs
- enabling the body to move
- production of heat
- storing calcium
- production of blood cells

· ·

Nursing Assistant/Nurse Aide Flash Review

DIAGNOSTIC TESTS FOR MUSCULOSKELETAL SYSTEM DISORDERS

. . . .

ABDUCTION

. . . .

ADDUCTION

Diagnostic tests for musculoskeletal system disorders include:

- Radiographs (X-rays) are used to detect fractures and other skeletal disorders.
- Nerve conduction studies measure the electrical activity of muscles when they contract and are used to determine whether the muscles and nerves are working properly.
- A muscle biopsy warrants the removal of a small piece of muscle to diagnose musculoskeletal abnormalities.
- Arthrocentesis involves the insertion of a needle into a disordered joint and removal of fluid to check for abnormal cells and bacteria.

. . . .

Abduction is moving away from the body's midline.

. . . .

Adduction is moving toward the body's midline.

AMPUTATIONS

. . . .

CAST CARE

. . . .

The removal of an arm or a leg is called an amputation. Causes include accidents, war injuries, and illnesses. Diabetes can lead to amputation when a person's toes or foot become gangrenous from impaired blood flow. Losing a body part is traumatic, both emotionally and physically, as it can affect a person's body image, mobility, and lifestyle. Stump (end of the amputated part) care is critical to allow for proper prosthetic fitting. The end of the stump will be wrapped to shrink and shape it, and range of motion exercises will be used to keep muscles and tendons from shortening. The stump will also be observed for signs of infection. Some people experience phantom pain or a sensation that the body part is still attached. This is caused by healing of the nerves at the end of the stump and usually disappears shortly after surgery.

• •

Casts are usually used for fractures, but may also be used for other problems. They can be made of plaster of paris or fiberglass.

When caring for a client in a cast, the nursing assistant will:

• Keep the casted body part elevated as ordered.

• Turn the client as ordered to allow the cast to dry.

• Not use fingertips when handling the cast (to prevent denting).

• Keep the cast clean and dry.

• Make sure the fingers or toes of the casted body part are warm, pink, and mobile.

• Report any complaints of pain, numbness, or tingling, as well as cyanosis, swelling, or coldness of the areas around the cast.

• Tell the client not to scratch the skin under the cast, even when itchy.

• Tell the client to avoid weight bearing on the cast.

• If walking on a cast is allowed, be sure to place the cast boot on before ambulation.

• Report any wetness, odor, or deterioration of the cast.

• •

Nursing Assistant/Nurse Aide Flash Review

DORSIFLEXION

. . . .

EFFECTS OF AGING ON THE MUSCULOSKELETAL SYSTEM

. . . .

EVERSION

Dorsiflexion is flexing the foot in an upward direction toward the knee.

· ·

The effects of aging on the musculoskeletal system include:

- aches, pain, and stiffness, as well as loss of strength and endurance
- changes in the musculoskeletal system (the leading cause of disability in older adults)
- decreased ability to absorb calcium, causing loss of bone tissue
- muscle atrophy (decreased size and strength)
- loss of flexibility in the joints due to loss of the proteins that normally make cartilage, ligaments, and tendons flexible

· ·

Eversion is rotating the sole of the foot outward.

EXTENSION

· ·

FLEXION

· ·

FRACTURES

PART 2

Extension is straightening a joint.

· ·

Flexion is bending a joint.

· ·

Fractures are breaks in the bone. They are usually caused by trauma, but can also be caused by repeated stress (stress fractures) or disease (pathological fractures). Older adults are at risk for fractures because their bones are fragile and they are susceptible to falls. Types of fractures include:

- Greenstick: bend or splintering of the bone, seen mostly in children.

- Closed (simple): broken bone does not protrude through the skin.

- Open (compound): broken bone protrudes through the skin, increasing the risk for infection.

- Spiral: winding break, usually caused by a twisting injury.

- Comminuted: the bone break area shatters into little pieces.

Fractures often require bringing the broken ends into alignment (reduction) and a manner to hold them together (fixation). When this process is performed without a surgical incision, it is called closed reduction, and when it is performed using surgical intervention, it is called open reduction.

HIP FRACTURES

. . . .

INADEQUATE MUSCULOSKELETAL FUNCTIONING

. . . .

INVERSION

Hip fractures are common in older adults, especially females. The fracture is a break at the top of the femur, and usually requires surgical reduction with the insertion of pins, plates, or screws, or replacement with an artificial hip joint. The prognosis for a hip fracture can be guarded, as a large number of older adults die shortly after the hip fracture.

. . . .

It is important that the nursing assistant observe for signs that a client is experiencing a musculoskeletal problem. These signs should be reported to the nurse immediately:

- redness, swelling, tenderness, or pain in the affected area
- coldness or paleness at an affected site
- pain when moving a joint
- decreased range of motion
- limping or refusal to walk
- guarding a joint or limb
- decreased muscle strength
- falls

. . . .

Inversion is rotating the sole of the foot inward.

MUSCULAR DYSTROPHY (MD)

. . . .

OSTEOARTHRITIS

. . . .

OSTEOPOROSIS

PART
2

MD is a group of inherited disorders where the muscles progressively weaken over time. The effects can be moderate to fatal, depending on the type of MD. Duchene's MD is the most common and most debilitating form of MD in children. It develops during early childhood and usually causes death by the time the child is 20 as the muscles required for breathing become unable to perform. In adults, myotonic MD is the most common form, which leads to heart and endocrine problems, and to cataracts.

. . . .

In caring for clients with joint replacements, nursing assistants will probably need to assist clients with transfers because they will not be able to bear weight on the affected joint for some time. Clients who have had hip replacements will need additional care, such as keeping their legs abducted by using an abduction or regular pillow, using a straight-backed chair for sitting, using a device to raise the toilet seat, and avoiding flexing the hips more than 90 degrees.

. . . .

Osteoporosis is excessive loss of bone that causes the bones to become very fragile and to break easily. Commonly affected bones include those in the spine, pelvis, arms, and legs. Risk factors include female gender, white race, older age, family history of osteoporosis, small body frame, smoking, and inactivity, as well as eating disorders, diet low in calcium, Vitamin D, and protein; excessive alcohol use; and certain medications, including steroids.

Nursing assistants should be careful when handling a person with osteoporosis during transfer. They should also monitor the client's dietary intake and watch for signs of fractures.

Nursing Assistant/Nurse Aide Flash Review

PLANTAR FLEXION

. . . .

PRONATION

. . . .

SUPINATION

Pantar flexion is flexing the foot in a downward direction.

. . . .

Pronation is rotating the palm to face upward (like carrying a tray).

. . . .

Supination is rotating the palm to face downward.

PART 2

STRUCTURE OF THE NERVOUS SYSTEM

. . . .

FUNCTIONS OF THE NERVOUS SYSTEM

. . . .

The nervous system includes the following components:

Central nervous system (CNS)

- Brain
    - Cerebrum (controls thinking, speaking, memory, emotions, voluntary muscle movement, sensory information interpretation).
    - Diencephalon (thalamus controls impulses from the spinal cord and sends them to the cerebrum; hypothalamus controls temperature, appetite, fluid balance, and some emotions; and epithalamus controls sleep cycles, sensory reception, temperature and fluid balance, and some endocrine functions).
    - Cerebellum (controls coordination and balance).
    - Brain stem (controls heartbeat, respirations, and blood pressure).
- Spinal cord
    - Maintains the connection between the brain and the body.

Peripheral nervous system (PNS)

- All nerves outside of the brain and spinal cord
- Somatic nervous system (voluntary)
    - Sensory (afferent) nerves (carry information from the organs to the spinal cord and to the brain).
    - Motor (efferent) nerves (carry commands from the brain to the spinal cord and to the organs).
- Autonomic nervous system (involuntary)
    - Sympathetic
        - Is activated by stress (fight or flight).
        - Increases heart rate, blood pressure, breathing rate, pupil size, sweating.
    - Parasympathetic
        - Maintains body functions; in control when relaxed.
        - Restores body to prestress state.

· ·

The functions of the nervous system are:

- regulating homeostasis
- activating responses to dangerous situations (fight or flight)
- allowing humans to interact with the world.

· ·

Nursing Assistant/Nurse Aide Flash Review

DIAGNOSTIC TESTS FOR NERVOUS SYSTEM DISORDERS

. . . .

CEREBRAL VASCULAR ACCIDENT (CVA)

. . . .

SYMPTOMS OF A STROKE

Diagnostic tests for nervous system disorders are:

- Electroencephalogram (EEG) measures the electrical activity of the brain and is used to check for a seizure disorder.

- Imaging studies such as computed tomography (CT) scan and magnetic resonance imaging (MRI) help locate tumors in the nervous system.

· ·

A cerebral vascular accident (CVA), also known as a stroke or brain attack, happens when the blood flow to part of the brain is blocked or interrupted. Most strokes are ischemic (severely reduced blood flow) and caused by either a clot forming (thrombotic stroke) in one of the brain arteries or a clot forming elsewhere (usually the heart), breaking off, and traveling to the brain. This is called an embolic stroke. Some strokes are caused by bleeding when a blood vessel in the brain leaks or ruptures; this can be caused by uncontrolled high blood pressure, an aneurysm (weak spot in a blood vessel), trauma, anticoagulant medication, or a bleeding disorder such as hemophilia.

· ·

Sudden severe headache; dizziness; loss of balance or coordination; slurred or garbled speech or difficulty understanding others; sudden blindness in one or both eyes or double vision; drooping of one side of the mouth; sudden weakness, numbness, or paralysis in the face, arm, or leg, usually on one side of the body. Symptoms vary according to the location of the stroke in the brain.

POSSIBLE LASTING EFFECTS OF A STROKE

. . . .

COMA

. . . .

- Memory loss: there may also be difficulty with reasoning and making judgments.

- Emotional difficulties: the client may have difficulty in controlling emotions or depression.

- Expressive aphasia: the client may have difficulty speaking and may also have difficulty swallowing, which increases the risk of choking.

- Receptive aphasia: there may be difficulty understanding words; the person can speak but may have trouble following directions.

- Loss of muscle movement: control may be lost over certain muscles, such as on one side of the face or arm.

- Hemiplegia: there may be paralysis of one side of the body.

A stroke is a medical emergency, and immediate treatment can help minimize permanent damage. Treatment may also include intensive care, respiratory support, and continuous monitoring. Clients can experience depression and frustration as a result of their sudden disabilities. Ongoing treatment depends on the extent of the damage, and this can create emotional and financial difficulties for the family, who may need to decide about home healthcare, long-term care, or discontinuing life support, depending on the client's condition.

. . . .

Coma is a state of unconsciousness in which the client cannot be awakened and cannot react to the surrounding environment. Comas can result from many causes, including stroke, brain tumors, hypothermia, drug overdoses, traumatic injuries, illnesses, near drowning, and choking. There are different levels of coma, and in the deepest level clients do not open their eyes, speak, or respond to pain with any body movement. The client is totally dependent for care.

. . . .

Nursing Assistant/Nurse Aide Flash Review

EFFECTS OF AGING ON THE NERVOUS SYSTEM

. . . .

EPILEPSY

. . . .

The effects of aging on the nervous system include:

- Reaction time is slowed due to decreased myelin and neurotransmitter imbalance, which can increase the risk of falls and other accidents.
- Memory for past events remains intact, but recall may slow; mild recent memory loss is possible.
- Sensory changes occur (visual, hearing, and taste perception alterations).
- Dementia is a disorder, not a normal aging process.

Exercising the mind helps preserve brain function. Therefore, the nursing assistant can encourage older clients to read, do crafts, work on puzzles, or engage in other activities that stimulate thinking and creativity.

· ·

Epilepsy is a chronic seizure disorder, and seizures are caused by disruptions in the normal electrical activity of the brain. The cause of epilepsy is usually unknown; however, seizures can be caused by heredity, and by problems that include head trauma, strokes, meningitis, AIDS, prenatal injuries, and developmental disorders. Common types of seizures are:

- absence seizures (petit mal): staring and subtle body movement, possible brief loss of awareness, rapid blinking
- tonic seizures: stiffening of the muscles, generally in the back, arms, and legs
- clonic seizures: rhythmic, jerking muscle contractions, usually in the neck, face, and arms
- myoclonic seizures: sudden brief jerks or twitches of the arms and legs
- atonic seizures: loss of normal muscle tone and sudden collapse
- tonic-clonic seizures (grand mal): loss of consciousness, body stiffening and shaking, occasionally loss of bladder control or tongue biting, and temporary loss of breathing
- simple focal (partial) seizures: changes in emotions or the senses, involuntary muscle movements, no loss of consciousness
- complex focal (partial) seizures: staring and nonpurposeful movements (chewing movements, walking in circles); altered awareness or consciousness; inability to respond to questions or directions

Most people with epilepsy are well controlled with medication and live normal lives.

Nursing assistants should report signs of seizure activity to the nurse and know how to respond when a seizure occurs.

· ·

HEAD TRAUMA

. . . .

INADEQUATE NERVOUS FUNCTIONING

. . . .

MULTIPLE SCLEROSIS

PART 2

Head traumas can range from minor injury to fatal injury and are a major cause of death and disability. Many are caused by motor vehicle accidents, falls, gunshot wounds, and war trauma. The level of disability depends on the location of injury and the extent of the damage, and may include seizures, paralysis, memory problems, and behavioral issues. Rehabilitation and care are individualized. Many young people in long-term care are there because of head trauma.

. . . .

It is important that the nursing assistants observe for signs that a client is experiencing a nervous problem. These signs should be reported to the nurse immediately:

• decrease in the person's level of consciousness

• seizure activity

• changes in speech or movement

. . . .

Multiple sclerosis (MS) is a potentially incapacitating disorder in which the body's immune system destroys the protective sheath (myelin) that covers nerves, resulting in interference in the communication between the brain, spinal cord; and other areas of the body. Symptoms depend on the location and amount of damage and may include fatigue, dizziness, vision loss, double vision, tingling and pain, slurred speech, numbness or weakness in one or more extremities, and heat sensitivity that can trigger or worsen symptoms. Some people with MS completely lose their ability to speak or walk. MS is difficult to diagnose in its early stages because the symptoms wax and wane. There is no cure, but there are treatments that can treat attacks, manage the symptoms, and slow down the progress of the disease. MS may cause a young person to need long-term care.

When caring for persons with MS, nursing assistants should:

• Help decrease clients' risk of injury by following the care plan.

• Provide range of motion exercises as ordered to prevent contractures.

• Report difficulties with urination and defecation.

• Provide comfort.

• Maintain the person's dignity.

PARAPLEGIA

. . . .

PARKINSON'S DISEASE

. . . .

PERSISTENT VEGETATIVE STATE

Paraplegia is paralysis that affects all or part of the trunk, legs, and pelvic organs.

. . . .

Parkinson's disease is a gradually progressive disorder of the nervous system that affects movement. It is caused by insufficient production of the neurotransmitter dopamine, which is necessary for the functioning of motor neurons. The brain's directions do not reach the muscles to control body movement. Symptoms include tremors, bradykinesia (slowed movement), muscle rigidity, impaired balance and posture, and speech and writing changes, as well as loss of automatic movements (smiling, blinking, swinging arms when walking). Parkinson's disease cannot be cured; however, there are medications that improve symptoms.

When caring for a client with Parkinson's disease, the nursing assistant should:

• Report increased symptoms to the nurse.

• Schedule personal care when the client is doing well.

• Possibly assist clients to speech and other therapies.

. . . .

A persistent vegetative state (PVS) exists when a person is awake, but totally unaware. The person can no longer relate meaningfully with the environment, recognize loved ones, or feel emotions or discomfort, because the higher levels of the brain no longer function. The person in a PVS has sleep/wake cycles and can cough, sneeze, scratch, and even cry or smile. The person may move the arms or legs and have automatic reactions to touch, sound, and light. However, these are automatic behaviors that do not require any functioning of the thinking part of the brain. The person in a PVS is totally dependent for care.

PART 2

QUADRIPLEGIA

. . . .

SPINAL CORD INJURIES

. . . .

TRANSIENT ISCHEMIC ATTACKS

Quadriplegia is paralysis of all four extremities, and often also includes bladder, bowel, and sexual dysfunction.

· ·

A spinal cord injury is damage to any part of the spinal cord. It is usually caused by trauma and often causes permanent damage in strength, sensation, and other body functions below the site of the injury. Disability depends on the location and severity of the injury and may include loss of movement and/or sensation; loss of bowel or bladder control; changes in sexual function, sexual sensitivity, and fertility; pain; and difficulty breathing, coughing, or clearing secretions. Care also depends on the extent of the disability. Clients who experience quadriplegia usually need total assistance, while clients with paraplegia may need little assistance after rehabilitation. Spinal cord injuries can also be emotionally devastating, and thus, clients and families need support and encouragement to engage in self-care and learn to give care to their loved one.

· ·

Transient ischemic attacks (TIAs) are brief episodes of decreased blood flow to a part of the brain. They can be caused by tiny blood clots that clog narrow arterioles. Risk factors include family history, age over 55, sickle cell disease, high blood pressure, cardiovascular disease, peripheral artery disease, diabetes, obesity, heavy drinking, illicit drug abuse, cigarette smoking, and birth control pills.

Symptoms of TIAs are dizziness, loss of balance or coordination, slurred or garbled speech or difficulty understanding others, or sudden blindness in one or both eyes or double vision, as well as sudden weakness, numbness, or paralysis in the face, arm, or leg, usually on one side of the body. Symptoms vary according to the location of the TIA in the brain. Symptoms last for minutes to several hours, but disappear within 24 hours.

TIAs are usually warning signs of a stroke, so if the nursing assistant suspects that a client is experiencing a TIA, the nursing assistant should report this immediately to the nurse.

PART 2

STRUCTURE OF THE SENSORY SYSTEM

· ·

FUNCTIONS OF THE SENSORY SYSTEM

· ·

DIAGNOSTIC TESTS FOR SENSORY SYSTEM DISORDERS

The sensory system consists of sensory receptors that pick up and translate information and send it to the brain for interpretation, as well as sensory organs (skin, tongue, nose, eyes, and ears).

- Tactile: The skin has tactile receptors (more in some areas than others) that respond to touch. There are also position receptors in the muscles, tendons, and joints that allow people to be aware of their body position, and pain receptors that signal distress.

- Taste: Taste organs are in the tongue. The four tastes are bitter, sweet, sour, and salty.

- Smell: Smell organs are in the roof of the nasal cavity. The sense of smell wears out easily, so bad odors become less noticeable with time.

- Sight: The structures of the eye include the pupil, iris, lens, retina, optic nerve, and macula.

- Hearing: The ear incudes the outer ear (pinna or auricle), the middle ear, and the inner ear.

· ·

The functions of the sensory system are:

- The senses allow people to experience their world.

- The senses allow people to feel, taste, smell, see, and hear.

- The ear also helps maintain balance.

· ·

Diagnostic tests for sensory system disorders include:

- Snellen chart is used to assess vision.

- Audiometer screening is used to assess hearing.

- Tuning fork tests are used to detect hearing loss.

CATARACTS

. . . .

CONJUNCTIVITIS

. . . .

CONTACT LENS CARE

PART 2

A cataract is clouding of the lens of the eye, making vision seem like looking though a fogged-up window. Other symptoms include increasing difficulty with night vision, sensitivity to light, seeing halos around lights, fading or yellowing of colors, and double vision. Eyeglasses may help initially; however, surgery is usually needed. This surgery is now simple and usually allows the client to go home that same day.

. . . .

Conjunctivitis (pink eye) is an inflammation of the conjunctiva that may be caused by irritation, allergy, or infection. When an infection is present, conjunctivitis is highly contagious.

. . . .

Contact lenses are plastic disks that fit directly on the eye to correct vision. They must be cleaned and stored properly to prevent damage to the contacts and the chance of infection. When caring for a person's contact lenses, the nursing assistant should also make sure to place each lens in its proper storage container, usually marked left and right, and use the proper solution.

Nursing Assistant/Nurse Aide Flash Review

DIABETIC RETINOPATHY

. . . .

EAR INFECTIONS

. . . .

EFFECTS OF AGING ON THE SENSORY SYSTEM

PART 2

Diabetic retinopathy is a complication of diabetes that can cause blindness because elevated blood sugar can affect the eye lenses and damage the blood vessels of the light-sensitive tissue in the retina. Persons may be asymptomatic at first, and then develop spots or floaters in their vision, blurred vision, difficulty with color perception, dark or empty areas in their vision, and vision loss.

· ·

Outer ear infections (otitis externa, swimmer's ear) is a painful inflammation that is common in swimmers. It is usually treated with eardrops. Middle ear infections (otitis media), which are common in children, are usually caused by bacteria and are treated with antibiotics.

· ·

The effects of aging on the sensory system include:

- clouding of the eye lenses
- rigidity of the iris that makes it take longer to adjust to light changes
- presbyopia, which is decreased near vision
- dry eye from decreased tear production
- presbycusis, which is the gradual loss of hearing of high-pitched sounds
- decreased taste and smell due to decreased receptors in the nose and tongue

EYEGLASS CARE

. . . .

GLAUCOMA

. . . .

HEARING AIDS

When caring for a person who wears eyeglasses, nursing assistants should:

• Make sure the client wears them when needed.

• Use caution when handling the glasses.

• Clean glasses with the proper solutions and cloths.

• Avoid cleaning glasses with napkins or paper towels, as these may scratch the lenses.

. . . .

Glaucoma is a group of eye conditions that results in optic nerve damage and possible loss of vision. It usually is caused by abnormally high pressure inside the eye (intraocular pressure).

Primary open-angle glaucoma, the most common type, has no noticeable signs or symptoms except gradual vision loss. However, glaucoma can also occur suddenly. When that happens, it is usually accompanied by severe pain. Risk factors include age over 40, African American ethnicity, heredity, other eye disorders, and long-term use of corticosteroids. Treatment includes eyedrops and/or surgery.

. . . .

Hearing aids are battery-operated devices that increase sound before it enters the auditory canal. They do not work for all types of hearing loss. They come in different styles: completely in the canal, in the canal, half shell, full shell, and behind the ear.

When caring for hearing aids, nursing assistants should:

• Clean them daily, according to the instructions.

• Replace dead batteries immediately.

• Make sure the client has spare batteries, and keep them away from children and pets.

• Avoid using hair-care products when the hearing aid is in use.

• Store hearing aides at room temperature.

HEARING LOSS

....

IMPACTED CERUMEN

....

INADEQUATE SENSORY FUNCTIONING

Hearing loss occurs gradually with age (presbycusis), but it can also be caused by heredity, built-up cerumen (earwax), exposure to loud noises, and trauma. It can be conductive (something prevents waves from reaching the receptors in the cochlea) or sensorineural (receptors are unable to receive or transmit nerve impulses). Hearing loss is not reversible; however, there are treatments that can improve hearing. These include removing cerumen, using hearing aids, and cochlear implants.

When caring for a person with hearing loss, the nursing assistant can use communication skills:

- Face the person when speaking.

- Write down important directions or questions.

- Get feedback to make sure the person understands.

- Let the person know if the nursing assistant cannot understand the person.

- Learn sign language.

- Use communication boards or cards available through speech therapy departments.

. . . .

Impacted cerumen (earwax) occurs when earwax builds up and causes decreased hearing. It is common in older adults and is usually treated with drops or irrigations.

. . . .

It is important that the nursing assistant observes for signs that a client is experiencing a sensory problem. These signs should be reported to the nurse immediately:

- pain

- sudden hearing loss

- sudden vision loss

Nursing Assistant/Nurse Aide Flash Review

MACULAR DEGENERATION

. . . .

MÉNIÈRE'S DISEASE

. . . .

PROSTHETIC EYE CARE

PART
2

Macular degeneration causes vision loss in the center of the field of vision. The cause is unknown, but deposits build up in the macula. Risk factors include heredity, age over 50, white race, smoking, obesity, diet low in fruits and vegetables, cardiovascular disease, and elevated cholesterol.

. . . .

Ménière's disease is a problem of the inner ear that causes vertigo (feeling like one is spinning), as well as tinnitus (ringing in the ear); feeling of pressure in the ears; and progressive hearing loss. The cause is not known, and it is most common in persons in their 40s and 50s. The problem can persist, and when an attack occurs, the person should lie down and keep the eyes fixed on a nonmoving object. Persons should also take their time getting up from a sitting or lying position to minimize attacks.

. . . .

An eye may be removed due to illness or injury, and the affected person may wear an artificial eye (prosthesis). Some are permanent and others are removable. If the eye is removable, the nursing assistant should help with cleaning and handle the prosthesis with care to prevent breakage by accidentally falling to the floor or other hard surface.

VISUAL IMPAIRMENT

· ·

Visual impairment may take many forms, including blindness. Blindness may be caused by heredity, disease, or trauma, and the affected person may see nothing, or may see some light, movement, shades, or colors. Most people adapt well and are independent, but they may need to learn how to navigate safely and read Braille. Some may also adapt with the use of a service animal.

When working with a person who is blind, the nursing assistant should:

- Find out the extent of the person's vision loss.

- Speak normally.

- Be descriptive of the surroundings.

- Tell the person when the nursing assistant enters the room and when the nursing assistant leaves.

- Explain procedures completely and descriptively.

- Avoid rearranging the furniture.

- Leave the door either open or closed, not in between.

- Walk with the person at the nursing assistant's side while holding the person's elbow, if assistance is needed.

STRUCTURE OF THE ENDOCRINE SYSTEM

. . . .

FUNCTIONS OF THE ENDOCRINE SYSTEM

. . . .

The endocrine system includes the following glands:

- Pituitary: lies underneath the brain.

- Pineal: lies underneath the brain.

- Thyroid: is located in the neck.

- Parathyroids: are located in back of the thyroid.

- Thymus: is located above the heart.

- Adrenals: are located on top of the kidneys.

- Pancreas: is located in the abdomen.

- Gonads: are the ovaries and testes.

. . . .

The functions of the endocrine system are:

- Pituitary: The posterior lobe of this master gland secretes antidiuretic hormone (ADH) that limits water excretion and oxytocin that stimulates labor and causes the let-down of breast milk in nursing mothers. The anterior lobe secretes growth hormone, thyroid-stimulating hormone (TSH), adrenocorticotropic hormone (ACTH) that stimulates the adrenals, prolactin (PRL) to stimulate breast milk production, and gonadotropins that regulate the function of the gonads.

- Pineal: This gland secretes melatonin that helps regulate the sleep/wake cycle.

- Thyroid: This secretes thyroxin to control metabolism and calcitonin to regulate calcium in the bloodstream.

- Parathyroids: These secrete parathyroid hormone, which has the opposite effect of calcitonin.

- Thymus: The thymus secretes thyroxin to fight infection.

- Adrenals: The medulla secretes epinephrine and norepinephrine for the fight or flight response. The cortex secretes glucocorticoids to help maintain glucose levels and to suppress the body's immune response, mineralocorticoids to help regulate certain minerals, and androgens that are converted to sex hormones.

- Pancreas: The pancreas secretes insulin to allow blood sugar into the cells, and glucagon that has the opposite effect.

- Gonads: The gonads secrete hormones that start puberty and regulate reproduction.

. . . .

Nursing Assistant/Nurse Aide Flash Review

DIAGNOSTIC TESTS FOR ENDOCRINE SYSTEM DISORDERS

. . . .

ACROMEGALY

. . . .

ADDISON'S DISEASE

. . . .

CUSHING'S DISEASE

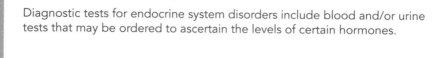

Diagnostic tests for endocrine system disorders include blood and/or urine tests that may be ordered to ascertain the levels of certain hormones.

. . . .

Acromegaly develops when the pituitary gland produces too much growth hormone during adulthood, usually during middle age. Symptoms include enlarged hands and feet; coarsened, enlarged facial features; coarse, oily, thickened skin; excessive sweating and body odor; fatigue, muscle weakness, pain, and limited joint mobility; menstrual cycle irregularities in women and erectile dysfunction in men; enlarged liver, heart, kidneys, spleen, and other organs; and increased chest size (barrel chest). Since this disorder progresses slowly, it may go unnoticed for years.

. . . .

Addison's disease occurs when the body produces insufficient amounts of the adrenal hormone cortisol and often aldosterone as well. It can occur at any age and may be life-threatening.

Symptoms include irritability, depression, fatigue, weight loss, decreased appetite, salt craving, body hair loss, darkening of the skin (hyperpigmentation), nausea and vomiting, diarrhea, and muscle weakness. Clients with Addison's disease may need assistance with walking, as well as range of motion exercises.

. . . .

Cushing syndrome occurs when the body is exposed to too much cortisol for a long period of time. While it can be caused by overproduction in the body, the most common cause of Cushing's disease is the use of oral corticosteroid medication. Symptoms include a rounded face, increased facial hair, fat deposits on the abdomen and between the shoulders, and pink or purple stretch marks on the skin. Cushing's can cause hypertension, bone loss, easy bruising, and, sometimes, diabetes.

DIABETES MELLITUS

Diabetes mellitus is a group of diseases that affect how the body uses blood glucose (blood sugar). The body cannot use glucose and thus, it builds up in the bloodstream, causing the person to experience fatigue, weakness, excessive thirst (polydipsia) and urination (polyuria), and blurred vision. Over time, diabetes can result in numerous problems, including blindness, cardiovascular disease, nerve damage, and kidney failure.

The types of diabetes mellitus are:

- Type 1 diabetes mellitus accounts for about 5% to 10% of all cases and is caused by destruction of the insulin-making cells of the pancreas, usually by the body's own immune system. Since these persons cannot make their own insulin, they must receive regular insulin injections to control their blood glucose.

- Type 2 diabetes mellitus is far more common and accounts for about 90% to 95% of all cases of diabetes. In this type of diabetes mellitus, the pancreas makes insulin, but the body cells do not respond to it. Risk factors include obesity and aging; however, it has become more common in younger people.

- Prediabetes is usually seen in people who are overweight and who have elevated glucose levels but are not yet diabetic. Lifestyle changes can delay or even prevent type 2 diabetes mellitus in these cases.

- Gestational diabetes is seen in some women during pregnancy. The placenta creates hormones that make cells more resistant to insulin. The pancreas normally responds by making more insulin; however, for those with gestational diabetes, it does not.

Diabetes mellitus is managed with medication, diet, and exercise. Medications include insulin for type 1 diabetes and oral medications for type 2. The diet should be balanced with limited fats and sweets, and it should be spread out over intervals during the day to maintain healthy blood sugar levels. Exercise helps lower glucose levels. Clients will also have to monitor their blood glucose levels regularly to assess for hypoglycemia and hyperglycemia. This is accomplished by using a glucometer that uses a drop of blood to calculate the glucose level. When assisting clients with monitoring their glucose levels, the nursing assistant should wear gloves.

When caring for a client with diabetes mellitus, the nursing assistant should report the following to the nurse immediately:

- signs of hyperglycemia or hypoglycemia
- food refusal
- taking food from others
- unknown gifts from family
- vomiting
- significant change in activity level

EFFECTS OF AGING ON THE ENDOCRINE SYSTEM

. . . .

HYPERGLYCEMIA

. . . .

HYPERTHYROIDISM

The effects of aging on the endocrine system include:

- Hormone production is decreased

- Secretion of hormones is slowed

- In females, menopause is the end of menstruation and the ability to bear children.

- In males, the hormone changes decrease the sex drive and function.

• •

Hyperglycemia is abnormally high blood sugar. Symptoms include:

- Early:
    - fatigue
    - headache
    - blurred vision
    - increased thirst (polydipsia)
    - frequent urination (polyuria)

- Late:
    - confusion
    - weakness
    - fruity-smelling breath
    - dry mouth
    - nausea and vomiting
    - shortness of breath
    - abdominal pain

These symptoms should be reported immediately to the nurse if the client is diabetic.

• •

Hyperthyroidism (overactive thyroid) results from overproduction of thyroxin. It can accelerate the metabolism considerably, causing significant symptoms: sudden weight loss although still eating, nervousness, anxiety, irritability, rapid heart rate, sweating, tremors, enlarged thyroid, thinning skin, and fine hair. Older adults have few or no symptoms, but may have subtle ones like heat intolerance and tiredness. Hyperthyroidism is treated with radiation or surgery.

Nursing Assistant/Nurse Aide Flash Review

HYPOGLYCEMIA

. . . .

HYPOTHYROIDISM

. . . .

Hypoglycemia is abnormally low blood sugar. Symptoms include:

- Early:
    - irritability
    - moodiness
    - anxiety
    - nervousness
    - headache
    - shakiness
    - dizziness
    - sweating
    - hunger
    - night sweats
    - nightmares

- Late/severe:
    - drowsiness
    - confusion
    - difficulty speaking or slurred speech
    - blurry or double vision
    - clumsiness
    - jerky movements
    - muscle weakness
    - seizures
    - unconsciousness

These symptoms should be reported immediately to the nurse if the client is diabetic.

. . . .

Hypothyroidism, which is more common in females and the elderly, results when the thyroid gland does not produce enough thyroxin. Symptoms include fatigue, depression, increased cold sensitivity, constipation, dry skin, unexplained weight gain, muscle weakness, heavy or irregular menstrual periods, thinning hair, or slowed heart rate. People with hypothyroidism are treated with oral thyroxin.

. . . .

INADEQUATE ENDOCRINE FUNCTIONING

. . . .

PITUITARY DWARFISM

. . . .

PITUITARY GIGANTISM

It is important that the nursing assistant observe for signs that a client is experiencing an endocrine problem. These signs should be reported to the nurse immediately:

- irritability

- sleepiness

- confusion

- high fever or abnormally low body temperature

- changes in heart or respiratory rate

- warm, moist skin

- sweating

- nausea

- vomiting

- diarrhea

- seizures

. . . .

Pituitary dwarfism, usually called acquired growth hormone deficiency or hypopituitarism, occurs when the body fails to make adequate growth hormone. The person is usually smaller than average, but normally proportioned. It is typically seen in childhood and treated with growth hormone.

. . . .

Pituitary gigantism occurs when the pituitary excretes too much growth hormone. The person is usually taller than average, but normally proportioned.

Nursing Assistant/Nurse Aide Flash Review

STRUCTURE OF THE HEMATOLOGICAL SYSTEM

. . . .

FUNCTIONS OF THE HEMATOLOGICAL SYSTEM

. . . .

DIAGNOSTIC TESTS FOR HEMATOLOGICAL SYSTEM DISORDERS

The hematological system includes the following components:

- Red blood cells, also called erythrocytes, are made in the red marrow.
- White blood cells, also called leukocytes, come in five types: neutrophils, basophils, eosinophils, monocytes, and lymphocytes.
- Platelets, also called thrombocytes, enable blood clotting.
- Plasma is the liquid portion of the blood and is made up of 90% water and 10% dissolved materials such as amino acids, glucose, and fats.

. . . .

The functions of the hematological system are:

- Red blood cells carry oxygen to the cells.
- White blood cells fight infection.
- Platelets enable blood clotting.

. . . .

Diagnostic tests for hematological system disorders include a complete blood count test that measures several components and features of the blood, including red blood cells, white blood cells, hemoglobin, hematocrit, and platelets.

Nursing Assistant/Nurse Aide Flash Review

ANEMIA

. . . .

BLEEDING DISORDERS

. . . .

EFFECTS OF AGING ON THE HEMATOLOGICAL SYSTEM

PART 2

The word *anemia* represents a group of disorders that affect the red blood cells and decrease the body's ability to transport oxygen to cells. Anemia can result from loss of red blood cells (bleeding), destruction of red blood cells (hemolysis), or decreased production of red blood cells. Anemia can also result when there are ample red blood cells but they do not contain adequate hemoglobin. Iron is needed to make hemoglobin, and people with iron deficiency can develop anemia. Other anemias develop because of abnormal hemoglobin. These include sickle cell anemia, where the cells "sickle" or turn into little hooks. This shape causes them to be oxygen and nutrient deficient and to hook onto each other and form clots that can cause organ damage. Thalassemia is another anemia whereby the hemoglobin is abnormal.

. . . .

Bleeding disorders can cause too little or too much clotting. Hemophilia is a bleeding disorder that can result in prolonged bleeding. For some of these clients, a small injury can have fatal consequences, especially if the bleeding occurs in the head. Other clients develop clots. A thrombus can decrease circulation where it lies. It can also break off and turn into an embolus and travel to vital organs, which can also be fatal. Clients who clot easily are placed on anticoagulant medications.

. . . .

Aging may affect the bone marrow and blood cells of the hematological system, which may result in anemia in older adults.

Nursing Assistant/Nurse Aide Flash Review

INADEQUATE HEMATOLOGICAL FUNCTIONING

. . . .

LEUKEMIA

. . . .

PART 2

It is important that the nursing assistant observe for signs that a client is experiencing a hematological problem.

• bleeding or bruising

• tiredness

• signs of infection

. . . .

Leukemia is a cancer of the white blood cells. The white blood cell count is high, but the cells do not function properly, causing the client to develop infections. Persons with leukemia also are at risk for bleeding due to low platelet count, and for fatigue from low red blood cell count. Therefore, these clients will need precautions taken to prevent these problems.

. . . .

Nursing Assistant/Nurse Aide Flash Review

Human Needs

MASLOW'S HIERARCHY OF NEEDS

. . . .

PHYSIOLOGICAL NEEDS

. . . .

SAFETY AND SECURITY NEEDS

Self-actualization (morality, creativity, spontaneity, lack of prejudice)

Esteem (confidence, achievement, respect of and by others)

Love/belonging (family, friends, sexual intimacy)

Safety (security of body, employment, resources, family, health, property)

Physiological (air, water, food, sleep, sex, homeostasis, excretion)

. . . .

These are the most basic needs, and they are critical for survival. Therefore, they take priority over the other needs.

- A person will die within minutes without oxygen.
- Water, food, and the elimination of body wastes are critical for survival.
- Physical activity and rest promote bodily functioning and rejuvenation and prevent wasting.
- Sexual activity allows humans to reproduce and prevent extinction.

Nursing assistants help clients with their basic needs in many ways, including assisting them with meals, ambulating, and toileting.

. . . .

Being safe and secure means both being and feeling safe. Nursing assistants, like other healthcare providers, follow policies and procedures to assure client safety. Security needs include:

- well-being
- financial security
- healthcare
- safe neighborhoods
- childproofing the house
- allowing as much control as possible

Nursing assistants routinely help clients with their safety and security needs: hand washing to prevent infection, assuring that bed rails are up to prevent falls, and helping clients to get their questions answered quickly. They also help by making sure the call bell is always within the client's reach.

LOVE/BELONGING NEEDS

. . . .

ESTEEM NEEDS

. . . .

SELF-ACTUALIZATION NEEDS

PART 3

Nursing assistants can help the client feel accepted and appreciated by using smiles, kind words, and a gentle touch, as well as by helping family members to feel comfortable at the client's facility to promote visitation.

. . . .

Esteem needs include self-esteem, self-respect, personal worth, social recognition, and accomplishment. Hospitalization can affect a client's self-esteem due to dependency on others, the physical effects of some illnesses, wearing a hospital gown, and becoming a number on an identification bracelet.

Nursing assistants can promote client esteem by respecting the client's values and beliefs, and by allowing clients to wear their own clothing and perform as many self-care tasks as possible.

. . . .

People who attain the highest level of Maslow's hierarchy have self-awareness, concern for their personal growth, and interest in fulfilling their full potential. For clients, personal growth may mean regaining basic abilities, like learning to talk and walk again after a stroke.

Nursing assistants play an important role in promoting self-actualization for their clients by helping them achieve their health goals, as well as for themselves by attaining professional goals.

Nursing Assistant/Nurse Aide Flash Review

ERIKSON'S EIGHT STAGES

· ·

ERIKSON'S STAGE FOR INFANTS

· ·

ERIKSON'S STAGE FOR TODDLERS

PART
3

1. trust versus mistrust (birth to 1 year)

2. autonomy versus shame and doubt (1 to 3 years)

3. initiative versus guilt (3 to 6 years)

4. industry versus inferiority (6 to 12 years)

5. identity versus role confusion (12 to 20 years)

6. intimacy versus isolation (20 to 30 years)

7. generativity versus stagnation (30 to 65 years)

8. ego integrity versus despair (65 years and above)

. . . .

The Erikson stage for infants (birth to 1 year) is trust versus mistrust.

- In this stage, the infant's significant other is the caretaking person.

- This sense of trust forms the foundation for all future stages.

- Infants who experience consistently delayed needs gratification will develop a sense of uncertainty, leading to mistrust of caregivers and the environment.

. . . .

The Erikson stage for toddlers (1 to 3 years) is autonomy versus shame and doubt.

- The toddler is ready to assert his or her budding sense of control, independence, and autonomy.

- The toddler often uses "no," even when meaning yes, to assert independence (negativistic behavior).

- A sense of shame and doubt can develop if the toddler is kept dependent in areas where he or she is capable of using newly acquired skills or if made to feel inadequate when attempting new skills.

ERIKSON'S STAGE FOR PRESCHOOLERS

· ·

ERIKSON'S STAGE FOR SCHOOL-AGE CHILDREN

· ·

ERIKSON'S STAGE FOR ADOLESCENTS

PART 3

The Erikson stage for preschoolers (3 to 6 years) is initiative versus guilt.

- Preschoolers are energetic, enthusiastic, and intrusive learners with active imaginations.

- Conscience (an inner voice that warns and threatens) begins to develop.

- Development of a sense of guilt occurs when the child is made to feel that his or her imagination and activities are unacceptable.

- Guilt, anxiety, and fear result when the child's thoughts and activities clash with parental expectations.

. . . .

The Erikson stage for school-age children (6 to 12 years) is industry versus inferiority.

- A child's sense of industry grows out of a desire for real achievement.

- The child engages in tasks and activities that he or she can carry through to completion.

- The child learns rules, how to compete with others, and how to cooperate to achieve goals.

- Social relationships with others become increasingly important sources of support.

- The child can develop a sense of inferiority stemming from unrealistic expectations or a sense of failing to meet standards set for him or her by others.

. . . .

The Erikson stage for adolescents (12 to 20 years) is identity versus role confusion.

- To an adolescent, development of who he or she is and where he or she is going becomes a central focus.

- The adolescent continues to redefine his or her self-concept and roles that he or she can play with certainty.

- The inability to develop a sense of who he or she is and what he or she can become results in role confusion and inability to solve core conflicts.

Nursing Assistant/Nurse Aide Flash Review

ERIKSON'S STAGE FOR YOUNG ADULTS

. . . .

ERIKSON'S STAGE FOR MIDDLE-AGED ADULTS

PART
3

. . . .

ERIKSON'S STAGE FOR OLDER ADULTS

The Erikson stage for young adults (20 to 30 years) is intimacy versus isolation.

- Young adults can enter relationships without losing their identity.
- Intimate bonds may be formed in a heterosexual or a homosexual relationship.
- Isolation or avoidance of intimacy may develop when a person has not established identity, settles for stereotyped relationships, or engages in false intimacy.
- An isolated person may be lonely and withdrawn.

. . . .

The Erikson stage for middle-aged adults (30 to 65 years) is generativity versus stagnation.

- Adults need to contribute to the next generation by raising children or by producing something to pass on.
- Generativity means sharing, giving, and contributing to others.
- Stagnation means boredom and a sense of emptiness.
- Adults facing stagnation are inactive, self-absorbed, and self-indulgent.

. . . .

The Erikson stage for older adults (65 years and above) is ego integrity versus despair.

- This is a time for reviewing life events, especially experiences, and realizing that these have been good.
- There are cherished memories.
- The person has a meaningful part in history.

The contented older adult does not fear death.

- Failure to achieve ego integrity results in despair, resentment, futility, hopelessness, and a fear of death.

INFANCY

. . . .

INFANT DEVELOPMENTAL TASKS

. . . .

INFANT DEVELOPMENTAL MILESTONES

Infancy ranges from birth to 1 year of age.

Infants are considered neonates up to age 28 days.

Growth and development are most rapid during infancy.

- -

- Achieve physiologic balance.
- Learn to adjust to other people.
- Learn to love and be loved.
- Develop system of communication.
- Learn to express and control feelings.
- Develop foundations for self-awareness.

- -

- rolling
- sitting
- walking
- cooing
- laughing
- saying first words

INFANT HEALTH

· ·

INFANT SAFETY CONCERNS

· ·

- Breast milk is the most desirable complete feeding for first six months.
- Commercially prepared iron-fortified formula is an acceptable alternative.
- Solids are not recommended before age 4 to 6 months.
- Weaning from breast or bottle to cup should be gradual.
- Honey should be discouraged as it may cause infant botulism.
- Sleep patterns vary among infants.
- Stool color and consistency depend on what the infant eats. For all infants, these qualities change with the introduction of solids.
  - Breast-fed infants: seedy, may have up to four or five per day.
  - Bottle-fed infants: color, consistency, and odor depend on formula. Infants who receive milk-based formula have yellow to brown, soft or formed stools.
- Urinary output averages 200 to 300 ml by the end of the first week of life with about 20 voids per day.
- Primary tooth eruption begins by 6 months of age.
- Breast and bottle should be discouraged during sleep to prevent nursing (bottle) caries.

• •

- falling off bed or down stairs
- aspiration of small objects
- poisoning from overdose of medication or ingestion of toxic household substances
- suffocation due to inadvertent covering of the nose and mouth, pressure on the throat or chest, prolonged lack of air (such as in a closed parked car), or strangulation from crib rails or cords
- burns from hot liquids or foods, scalding bathwater, excessive sun exposure, or electrical injury
- motor vehicle accidents, most commonly linked to improper use or nonuse of infant car seat

• •

TODDLERHOOD

. . . .

TODDLER DEVELOPMENTAL TASKS

. . . .

TODDLER DEVELOPMENTAL MILESTONES

The toddler period is from age 1 to 3 years.

Physical growth is slow, but motor development increases.

Known for the "terrible twos," this is a time when children learn to be independent and when they have difficulty following rules.

· ·

- same as infants, plus:
- learning self-control
- toilet training

· ·

walking without help

scribbling

building block towers

saying about 300 words by age 2

primary dentition (20 deciduous teeth) usually completed by 2½ years

TODDLER HEALTH

. . . .

TODDLER SAFETY CONCERNS

. . . .

PRESCHOOL AGE

- Growth rate slows dramatically, thus decreasing the need for calories, protein, and fluids.
- Tantrums may be used to assert independence and are best dealt with by ignoring them or distracting the child.
- Negativism is also common, and the best way to decrease the number of "nos" is to decrease the number of questions that can lead to a "no" response.
- Sleep problems are common and may be due to fears of separation.
- Bedtime rituals and transitional objects, such as a blanket or stuffed toy, are helpful.
- By 12 months, most toddlers are eating the same foods as the rest of the family.
- At 18 months many become picky eaters, experiencing food jags and eating large amounts one day and very little the next.
- Toddlers are at risk for aspirating small food items such as peanuts.
- Readiness for toilet training does not usually occur until 18 to 24 months.
- Bowel training usually occurs before bladder training.

· ·

- Toddlers are prone to the same injuries as infants, as well as drowning.
- Caretakers need to remove unsafe objects from the toddler's reach.

· ·

The preschool period is age 3 to 6 years.

Preschoolers are adventurous and love to ask "why."

PRESCHOOL DEVELOPMENTAL TASKS

. . . .

PRESCHOOL DEVELOPMENTAL MILESTONES

. . . .

PRESCHOOL HEALTH

- Develop healthy routines.
- Become a participating family member.
- Learn to master impulses and conform to social expectations.
- Develop healthy emotional expressions.
- Learn effective communication.
- Develop ability to handle potentially dangerous situations.
- Develop initiative.
- Begin to learn that one's life has a purpose.

. . . .

- Can run, skip, and hop.
- Can tie shoes and copy a square by age 4.
- Can say 900 words by age 3.
- Knows four or more colors and the days of the week by age 5.

. . . .

- Four-year-olds are picky eaters.
- Five-year-olds are influenced by food habits of others.
- Sleep problems are common.
- Nightmares: the child can recall a frightening dream.
- Night terrors: the child appears fearful during sleep, but does not recall dream.
- Most children are capable of independent toileting by the end of the preschool period.
- The child needs regular interaction with same-age mates to help develop social skills.

PRESCHOOL SAFETY CONCERNS

. . . .

SCHOOL AGE

. . . .

SCHOOL-AGE DEVELOPMENTAL TASKS

- Preschoolers are somewhat less accident prone than toddlers, but they are still at risk for the same types of injuries and require many of the same types of safety precautions.

- Parents and other caretakers should emphasize safety measures, because preschoolers listen to adults and can understand and heed precautions.

- Preschoolers are great observers and imitate adults, so parents and other caretakers need to practice what they preach regarding safety.

• •

School age is 6 through 12 years.

School age is a period when children experience growth spurts, seek friendships, begin to think logically, and learn to play by the rules.

• •

- Learn basic knowledge and skills required for school.
- Master money management.
- Become an active family member.
- Extend abilities to relate to others.
- Manage feelings and impulses.
- Identify sex role.
- See self as worthy.
- Develop conscience and morality.

SCHOOL-AGE DEVELOPMENTAL MILESTONES

. . . .

SCHOOL-AGE HEALTH

. . . .

- bicycling, roller-skating, in-line skating, skateboarding; progressively improved running and jumping
- printing in early years; script in later years
- greater dexterity for crafts and video games
- computer competence
- development of various mental classifying and ordering activities

. . . .

- Caregivers should continue to stress the need for a balanced diet.
- The child is exposed to broader eating experiences in the school lunchroom.
- School-age children's individual sleep requirements vary but typically range from eight to nine hours per night.
- Beginning around age 6, permanent teeth erupt, and deciduous teeth are gradually lost.
- The child becomes increasingly involved in more complex activities, decisionmaking, and goal-directed activities.
- Peer relationships gain new importance.

. . . .

Nursing Assistant/Nurse Aide Flash Review

SCHOOL-AGE SAFETY CONCERNS

. . . .

ADOLESCENCE

. . . .

- A school-age child learns to accept more responsibility for personal health care and injury prevention.

- School-age children who learn safe swimming and diving practices, fire safety, use of seat belts and bicycle helmets, and other safety practices are at reduced risk for injury.

- The child's developing thinking skills aid in good judgment to avoid many types of injuries.

- School-age children are still prone to accidents, however, mainly due to increasing motor abilities and independence (e.g., a bicycle can take a child farther from home on his or her own).

- Major sources of injuries include bicycles, skateboards, and team sports. Learning proper techniques, using safety equipment, and, in the case of organized sports, receiving good coaching and playing with children of similar size can reduce the risk of injury.

- Parents should continue to provide guidance for new situations and threats to safety.

- The child should receive education about the use and abuse of alcohol, tobacco, and other drugs.

· ·

Adolescence is the period from 12 through 20 years.

Technically, adolescence begins at puberty, when secondary sex characteristics (e.g., breasts, pubic hair) begin to develop.

This is a stage of considerable growth and development, second only to infancy.

· ·

Nursing Assistant/Nurse Aide Flash Review

ADOLESCENT DEVELOPMENTAL TASKS

. . . .

ADOLESCENT DEVELOPMENTAL MILESTONES

. . . .

ADOLESCENT HEALTH

- Accept physical changes.
- Achieve satisfying and socially acceptable role.
- Develop more mature peer relationships.
- Achieve emotional independence.
- Get an education.
- Prepare for married or single life.
- Develop knowledge and skills for community relationships.
- Establish identity as a socially responsible person.

. . . .

- The young person develops abstract reasoning.
- Motor skills reach an adult level.

. . . .

Healthy diet may be difficult because of busy schedule, peers, and easy availability of fast foods.

Female adolescents are very prone to negative dieting behaviors.

Daily intake should be balanced among the foods in the pyramid and at www.choosemyplate.gov.

During adolescence, rapid growth, overexertion in activities, and a tendency to stay up late commonly interfere with sleep and rest requirements.

Many adolescents must wear orthodontic appliances, which may be a source of embarrassment.

Adolescents must pay special attention to careful brushing and care of teeth.

This period of rebellion and uncertainty can resemble the toddler period in certain respects.

Peer relationships become all-important for advice and support.

ADOLESCENT SAFETY CONCERNS

. . . .

YOUNG ADULTHOOD

. . . .

- Adolescents commonly are risk takers and often do not consider safety before action due to their feelings of invulnerability.
- Adolescents contribute substantially to motor vehicle accidents.
- Adolescents also are prone to accidents from unsafe use of bicycles, skateboards, motorcycles, boats, all-terrain vehicles, and snowmobiles.
- Accidental injury can result from improper use of firearms.
- Adolescents are particularly prone to swimming and diving accidents.
- Safety teaching should also reinforce the need for proper respect for gasoline, electricity, and fire.
- Adolescents need instruction on preventing sports injuries (e.g., avoiding overexertion, using proper equipment, techniques for making proper plays).
- Use of sunscreen during sun exposure should be encouraged.
- Smoking and use of alcohol and other drugs should be discouraged.
- Problem solving techniques should be taught to decrease use of physical violence as a coping mechanism.

. . . .

Young adulthood is the stage from 20 to 30 years.

Young adults typically enjoy the stability of a healthy life, but some may also still experience some of the issues of adolescence.

. . . .

YOUNG ADULT DEVELOPMENTAL TASKS

. . . .

YOUNG ADULT DEVELOPMENTAL MILESTONES

. . . .

YOUNG ADULT HEALTH

- Establish independence from parents.
- Establish household.
- Begin career or vocation.
- Develop personal lifestyle.
- Establish intimate relationship.
- Establish friendship network.
- Participate in community activities.
- Develop parenting behaviors.
- Implement personal values.

· ·

- time of optimal cognitive functioning
- engagement in mastery of new skills and knowledge
- intellect stimulated by exciting and challenging events

· ·

- Good nutrition is essential to physical fitness.
- Fatigue may be induced by physical work, inactivity, or stress.
- Ulcers and colitis can develop due to stress.
- Periodontal disease (gum disease) may begin to develop.
- Adult relationships are more enduring than earlier relationships.

Nursing Assistant/Nurse Aide Flash Review

YOUNG ADULT SAFETY CONCERNS

. . . .

MIDDLE AGE

. . . .

MIDDLE-AGE DEVELOPMENTAL TASKS—EARLY

PART 3

- safety precautions to prevent work-related injuries
- safety precautions to prevent sports- or exercise-related injuries

· ·

Middle adulthood is the period between 30 and 65 years.

This is a period of productivity or a time for more leisure. But it can also become the "sandwich" stage, when adults are faced with caring for both children and elderly parents.

· ·

- Adjust to changes of aging.
- Continue personal and professional interests.
- Review, refine, and evaluate career goals.
- Reach level of achievement.
- Work on maturing relationship.
- Choose organizational activities.
- Help young people develop.
- Develop leisure activities.
- Plan for retirement.

MIDDLE-AGE DEVELOPMENTAL TASKS—LATE

. . . .

MIDDLE-AGE DEVELOPMENTAL MILESTONES

. . . .

MIDDLE-AGE HEALTH

PART 3

- Develop supportive, interdependent relationships with children.
- Enhance relationship with significant other.
- Maintain community affiliations.
- Maintain interest in what's happening in the world.
- Develop satisfying leisure activities.
- Prepare for or adapt to retirement.
- Adapt to the changes of aging.

· ·

- Learning continues during adulthood.
- Reaction time and speed of intellectual performance are individual and stay the same or diminish during late middle age.
- Problem solving ability remains intact through adulthood; past experience is used to evaluate current situations.
- Memory generally remains intact; some decrease in recent memory may occur in late middle years.
- Creativity continues and may even increase.

· ·

- Regular physical activity increases life expectancy and life quality. It can also help prevent and manage coronary artery disease, hypertension, diabetes, osteoporosis, and depression.
- For each decade after 25 years of age, there should be a reduction in calories intake proportionate to activity level.
- Chronic health problems may begin.
- Many do not get adequate dental care.
- Oral cancers can go undetected.

MIDDLE-AGE SAFETY CONCERNS

. . . .

OLDER ADULTHOOD

. . . .

PART
3

OLDER ADULT DEVELOPMENTAL TASKS

- The major risk factors are environmental and behavioral.
- Preventive health screening for the following:
  - smoking behavior
  - alcohol use
  - obesity
  - heart disease and stroke
  - high cholesterol
  - cancers
  - sexually transmitted infections (STIs)
  - glaucoma

. . . .

Older adulthood is the period from 65 years forward.

Older adults may encounter chronic illness, decreased strength, and diminished senses.

. . . .

- Maintain self-image and sense of worth.
- Develop new family roles.
- Adjust to retirement.
- Adapt to physical changes.
- Adjust to satisfactory living arrangements.
- Work on life review.
- Prepare for own death.

Nursing Assistant/Nurse Aide Flash Review

OLDER ADULT DEVELOPMENTAL MILESTONES

. . . .

PART
3

OLDER ADULT HEALTH

. . . .

- There are few predictable changes in intellectual functioning.
- No decrease in general knowledge occurs.
- Increased wisdom may come with advancing age.
- Speed in mental performance and decisionmaking may slow.
- Mental functioning maintenance is affected by:
  - personal motivation
  - interest in the subject
  - sensory function
  - educational accomplishments
  - recentness of learning
  - personal value placed on intellectual activities

. . . .

- Exercise increases range of motion.
- Physical immobility hastens the aging process.
- Sufficient water/fluid intake is needed.
- Rest is important, with frequent rest periods and activity pacing recommended.
- Insomnia is common.
- Bladder volume capacity decreases.
- Bowel motility decreases.
- Medications, diet, and lack of exercise all contribute to elimination problems.
- Tooth decay, tooth loss, degeneration of the jawbone, gum recession, decreased saliva, and decreased thirst can affect appetite and digestion.
- Role changes occur with the deaths of loved ones.
- There has been a sharp rise in grandparents raising grandkids.
- Retirement can be positive or negative.

. . . .

OLDER ADULT SAFETY CONCERNS

. . . .

Older adults are vulnerable to falls and injuries to their integumentary and musculo-skeletal systems. Preventative measures include:

- Install padding on hard edges of wheelchairs and sharp surfaces.
- Pad arms of chairs.
- Wear gloves when washing dishes and gardening.
- Wear long sleeves to protect arms.
- Wear long pants to protect legs.
- Work and walk slowly to avoid collisions.
- Secure carpeting and throw rugs.
- Lower hot water temperature.

Nursing Assistant/Nurse Aide Flash Review

FAMILY FUNCTIONS

. . . .

FAMILY STRUCTURES

. . . .

POSSIBLE FAMILY RESPONSES TO ILLNESS AND HOSPITALIZATION

- childbearing and child rearing
- providing basic needs: food, safety, clothing, shelter, and healthcare
- providing communication and emotional support
- enabling enculturation and socialization
- preparing children to become citizens

. . . .

- nuclear or traditional
- single-parent
- reconstituted or blended
- extended
- same-sex
- two-career
- commuter
- return to nest
- binuclear (divorced parents assume joint custody)
- communal
- foster

. . . .

- fear and anxiety
- a sense of helplessness
- denial
- guilt
- anger
- frustration
- depression
- displacement
- projection

Nursing Assistant/Nurse Aide Flash Review

SEXUALITY

. . . .

SEX

. . . .

INTIMACY

PART 3

Sexuality is the way people view their maleness or femaleness. Sexuality can be affected by culture, religious beliefs, family values, and other influences, including illness. At times, persons' feelings about their sexuality do not match their physical makeup. A transsexual identifies himself or herself as a member of the opposite sex, and some of them have surgery and hormonal treatment to become that gender.

. . . .

Sex is physical activities that people engage in to experience pleasure or reproduce. The word *sex* is also used to denote one's gender.

. . . .

Intimacy is the feeling of emotional closeness to another.

Nursing Assistant/Nurse Aide Flash Review

SEXUAL ORIENTATION

. . . .

SEXUAL NEEDS OF OLDER ADULTS

. . . .

PART
3

Sexual orientation or preference denotes an enduring pattern of emotional, romantic, and/or sexual attraction.

- Heterosexuals are attracted to the opposite sex.
- Homosexuals are attracted to the same sex.
- Bisexuals are attracted to both sexes.

Sexual orientation also refers to the individual's sense of identity as based on those attractions.

. . . .

Sexual activity at any age is associated with circumstances, including an available partner. These circumstances strongly affect the elderly.

- The level of sexual activity for older women is directly related to their marital status. Throughout life, men are more sexually active than women.
- Chronic illness has a negative impact on sexual activity.
- Medication may also impair sexual activity.
- The level of sexual interest does not decrease with age.
- Decrease in sexual activity is not attributed to age, but to circumstances and illness.
- Older adults in long-term care facilities may find a new intimate partner while in the facility.

. . . .

Nursing Assistant/Nurse Aide Flash Review

NURSING ASSISTANT ROLE IN ASSISTING CLIENTS IN THEIR SEXUALITY NEEDS

. . . .

PART 3

- being nonjudgmental
- allowing for privacy
- always knocking before entering a room
- being aware that different cultures have different ideas about sexuality, and some are very concerned about their privacy and will not want to discuss sexual matters
- assisting clients to feel better about their sexuality (hair care, makeup, aftershave)
- redirecting a client who is masturbating in a public place (which may happen when a client is confused) to a more private location
- excusing self and quietly leaving if walking in on clients who are engaging in consensual sexual encounters in a private area

. . . .

Nursing Assistant/Nurse Aide Flash Review

CULTURE

. . . .

BELIEFS

. . . .

CUSTOMS

Culture is the learned values, beliefs, and customs of a designated group that are usually transmitted through the generations and that can influence one's thinking and behaviors.

Culture extends beyond ethnicity and religion to include aspects such as gender (e.g., lesbian, gay, transsexual, and bisexual [LGTB]), situation (e.g., prison culture), and location (e.g., rural), and it encompasses an array of values, beliefs, and customs.

. . . .

Beliefs are the opinions, knowledge, and faith about various aspects of the world.

. . . .

Customs are the learned behaviors that one can easily assess through observation and direct questioning.

VALUES

· ·

CULTURAL DIVERSITY

· ·

NURSING ASSISTANT ROLE IN ASSISTING CLIENTS IN THEIR CULTURAL NEEDS

PART 3

Values are the foundations for beliefs, attitudes, and behaviors

. . . .

Cultural diversity stands for the variety of cultures, races, ethnicities, and religions in the world.

- More than 30% of Americans are African American, Hispanic, Latino, or Asian.

- Latin Americans are the largest minority in the United States.

- A growing number of individuals belong to more than one race.

. . . .

- understanding their own culture

- learning about other cultures

- respecting and accepting people's differences, including those of co-workers, but not assuming differences or the lack of them

- being sensitive to nonverbal cues

- being sensitive to and accommodating cultural practices whenever possible and not harmful to health

SPIRITUALITY

. . . .

SPIRITUAL BELIEFS

. . . .

PART
3

SPIRITUAL CUSTOMS

Spiritual wellness involves the capacity for compassion, love, selflessness, forgiveness, joy, and fulfillment. Spirituality is a common bond between people. Some people look to organized religions to develop spiritual health, whereas others find meaning and purpose in their lives on their own through meditation, nature, art, or good works.

. . . .

Beliefs include opinions, knowledge, and faith about the world. Spiritual beliefs can range from atheism (belief that there is no God) to agnosticism (belief that God's existence is unknown or unknowable) to theism (belief that God is perfect and the creator of the universe). Beliefs, faith, and values interconnect—what one sets one's heart on, believes in, or lives out is what one values.

. . . .

Expressions of spirituality tend to follow an established order of practices, usually through a specific religious group. Practices range from simple meditation and relaxation to church services and rituals at shrines. Observances may take place at home with the family. Some traditions involve special foods or ceremonies on specific holy days, and these celebrations hold symbolic meaning and a deep sense of spirituality for those who follow the practices. Most religions have rituals to celebrate life stages, such as birth, entrance into adulthood, and death.

Nursing Assistant/Nurse Aide Flash Review

SPIRITUAL DISTRESS

. . . .

NURSING ASSISTANT ROLE IN ASSISTING CLIENTS IN THEIR SPIRITUAL NEEDS

. . . .

PART 3

Spiritual distress may be related to the inability to practice spiritual rituals, a conflict between spiritual beliefs and other aspects of life, or the crisis of illness, suffering, or death. Other definitions identify spiritual distress with unmet desires for support, compassion, and knowledgeable caring, as well as unmet needs for forgiveness, love, hope, and trust, and as an individual's inability to reach beyond the concerns of the self.

. . . .

- respecting clients' spiritual differences
- helping clients have time for their spiritual needs if desired and possible
- informing the nurse if factors impede the client's spiritual needs (e.g., taboo foods accidentally served at mealtime)

. . . .

The Nursing Assistant Role

TYPES OF HEALTHCARE SETTINGS

. . . .

ORGANIZATIONAL STRUCTURE

. . . .

PART
4

NURSING PERSONNEL

Nursing assistants will be employed in one of a number of healthcare agencies:

- Hospitals are institutions that provide a variety of treatments, including inpatient care. Clients are usually referred to as patients.

- Skilled nursing facilities are sub-acute-care facilities that usually provide rehabilitation.

- Long-term care facilities, also called nursing homes, provide care for people who cannot care for themselves but who do not need hospitalization. Clients are usually referred to as residents.

- Assisted-living facilities are for people who need some assistance with their daily care.

- Home healthcare agencies provide a variety of skilled healthcare needs to people in their own homes.

- Hospice provides care for people who are dying.

• •

Most agencies are governed by a board of trustees or board of directors that is made up of community members. The facility is managed by a chief executive officer (CEO). The next level of management is the directors (director of nursing, etc.), and each of these oversees their departments.

• •

According to the Bureau of Labor Statistics:

- Registered nurses (RNs) provide and coordinate client care, and educate clients and the public about various health conditions. They also provide advice and emotional support to clients and their family members.

- Licensed practical nurses (LPNs) or licensed vocational nurses (LVNs), depending on the state in which they work, provide basic nursing care. They work under the direction of registered nurses.

- Nursing assistants (nurse aides) help provide basic care for patients in hospitals and residents of long-term care facilities, such as nursing homes, as well as provide personal care in the home setting on an intermittent basis.

NURSING PROCESS

....

NURSING CARE MODELS

....

The nursing process is the center of holistic, client-focused care.

- Assessment: This is the collection and analysis of the client's physiological, psychological, sociocultural, spiritual, economic, and lifestyle data.

- Diagnosis: The nursing diagnosis is based on the client's response to actual or potential health conditions or needs.

- Outcomes and planning: These are short-term and long-term goals for the client's care.
    - Implementation: The nursing team carries out the plan.
    - Evaluation: The nursing team evaluates the effectiveness of the plan and modifies it as needed.

. . . .

Primary nursing is where one nurse is responsible for a group of clients.

- Modular or functional nursing is where each team member carries out the same task for each client.

- Team nursing is where the RN delegates tasks to each of the team members.

- Partners in practice is where care is delivered by a nurse partnering with a nursing assistant.

- Client-centered nursing is designed to meet each client's needs more effectively.

. . . .

Nursing Assistant/Nurse Aide Flash Review

OTHER HEALTHCARE TEAM MEMBERS

. . . .

REGULATORY AGENCIES

. . . .

PART 4

MANAGED CARE

- physicians
- nurse-practitioners
- clinical nurse specialists
- nurse-midwives
- nurse-anesthetists
- physician assistants
- physical therapists
- occupational therapists
- respiratory therapists
- nutritionists

. . . .

- The Joint Commission accredits and certifies healthcare organizations and programs in the United States. Accreditation and certification are recognized as a symbol of quality that reflects an organization's commitment to meeting certain performance standards.
- State boards of nursing are governmental agencies that are responsible for the regulation of nursing practice.

. . . .

Managed care plans contract with healthcare providers and medical facilities to provide care for members at reduced costs. There are three types:

1. A health maintenance organization (HMO) typically pays only for care within its network, although members can choose a primary care provider.

2. A preferred provider organization (PPO) typically pays more if the member obtains care within the network, but pays only a portion if the member goes outside the network.

3. Point of service (POS) plans let members choose either an HMO or a PPO each time they need care.

MEDICAID AND MEDICARE

. . . .

OMNIBUS BUDGET RECONCILIATION ACT (OBRA) OF 1987

. . . .

PART
4

NURSING ASSISTANT RESPONSIBILITIES

Medicaid and Medicare are government programs that provide health services to specific groups of people in the United States.

• Medicaid is for certain individuals and families with low incomes and few resources.

• Medicare is for elderly and certain disabled Americans.

· ·

The major purpose of OBRA of 1987 was to improve care for persons living in long-term care facilities. To assure that nursing assistants have the knowledge and skills to give quality care, OBRA requires that they complete a training program and pass a test before being employed in long-term care facilities.

· ·

Nursing assistants are responsible for meeting the basic needs of clients: hygiene, safety, comfort, nutrition, exercise, elimination, and emotional needs.

NURSING ASSISTANT QUALITIES

....

DELEGATION

....

PART 4

Nursing assistants should possess the following qualities:

- proper personal hygiene and appearance
- intrapersonal skills
- problem solving abilities
- time management skills
- goal setting skills
- stress management skills
- ethics

· ·

Delegation is passing of responsibility to another person (normally from a manager to a subordinate) to carry out specific activities.

The nurse must consider the following when delegating: the right task, the right circumstance, the right person, the right direction, and the right supervision.

· ·

Nursing Assistant/Nurse Aide Flash Review

PATIENTS' RIGHTS

. . . .

RESIDENTS' RIGHTS

PART 4

. . . .

CONFIDENTIALITY

The American Hospital Association's Patients' Bill of Rights has been replaced by the Patient Care Partnership that tells clients what to expect during their hospital stay:

- high-quality hospital care

- a clean and safe environment

- involvement in client care

- protection of client privacy

- help when leaving the hospital

- help with billing concerns

· ·

According to Medicare, nursing home residents' rights usually include:

- Respect: Residents have the right to be treated with dignity and respect.

- Services and fees: Residents must be informed in writing about services and fees before entering the nursing home.

- Money: Residents have the right to manage their own money or to choose someone else they trust to do this for them.

- Privacy: Residents have the right to privacy, and to keep and use their personal belongings as long as doing so does not interfere with the rights, health, or safety of others.

- Medical care: Residents have the right to be informed about their medical condition and medications, and the right to see their own doctor. They also have the right to refuse medications and treatments.

· ·

Confidentiality is the right of the client to have personal information kept private. Medical information, both verbal and written, should be available only to healthcare and insurance personnel as necessary.

HEALTH INSURANCE PORTABILITY AND ACCOUNTABILITY ACT (HIPAA)

. . . .

INFORMED CONSENT

. . . .

PART 4

ADVANCE DIRECTIVE

The Health Privacy Rule of the Health Insurance Portability and Account-ability Act (HIPAA) of 1996 protects the privacy and security of individual health data and establishes accountability and penalties for failing to use the rule to protect health information privacy.

. . . .

Informed consent is an agreement between a client and a physician that results in the client's authorization or agreement to undergo a specific medical intervention. Informed consent usually includes the diagnosis, nature, and purpose of the proposed treatment or procedure; risks and benefits of the proposed treatment or procedure; alternatives to the pro-posed treatment or procedure and their risks and benefits; and the risks and benefits of not undergoing the proposed treatment or procedure.

. . . .

Advance directives are legal documents that allow clients to legally specify their decisions about end-of-life care.

Nursing Assistant/Nurse Aide Flash Review

CIVIL LAW VIOLATIONS

. . . .

CRIMINAL LAW VIOLATIONS

. . . .

PART
4

ABUSE

Civil law violations (torts) include:

- slander: verbally making untrue statements about a person that harm that person's reputation
- libel: writing untrue statements about a person that harm that person's reputation
- fraud: deception that causes harm to another person
- false imprisonment: holding someone against that person's will
- invasion of privacy: breaching confidentiality or HIPAA

. . . .

- assault: threatening another person and causing someone to fear bodily harm
- battery: touching another person without his or her consent
- larceny: stealing
- abuse

. . . .

Types of abuse include:

- Physical abuse is the intentional use of physical force that may result in bodily injury and/or pain.
- Neglect, the most common form of abuse, is the refusal of a caretaker to provide the client with adequate food, water, clothing, and medical attention.
- Psychological abuse is the emotional abuse of a client through the infliction of verbal actions, including insults and humiliation.
- Financial abuse is the illegal or improper use of a client's property or funds.
- Sexual abuse is nonconsensual sexual contact.

Nursing Assistant/Nurse Aide Flash Review

PROFESSIONAL ETHICS

. . . .

PART 4

The Certified Nursing Assistant Code of Ethics and Conduct mandates that certified nursing assistants consider the emotional, physical, social, and spiritual needs of each patient:

- preserve life

- practice good health

- treat patients equally

- maintain confidentiality

- commit to continuing education

· ·

Nursing Assistant Skills

TYPES OF ORGANISMS

. . . .

INFECTIOUS DISEASE

. . . .

PART 5

Microorganisms or microbes are small living things, and some cannot be seen with the human eye. They include the following:

- Bacteria are typically one-celled organisms that live in colonies and cause numerous types of infections.
    - Cocci are round bacteria.
    - Bacilli are rod-shaped bacteria.
    - Spirilla are spiral-shaped bacteria.
    - Aerobic bacteria need air to survive.
    - Anaerobic bacteria die if in oxygen.
- Viruses, the smallest organisms, are bundles of protein.
- Fungi include yeasts and molds.
- Parasites include insect and worms that live on or in hosts and cause illness.

. . . .

An infectious (communicable) disease is an illness caused by an agent such as a bacterium or virus that can be transmitted from one person to another. Examples are AIDS, the flu, giardia, and gonorrhea. Infectious diseases include:

- contact-transmitted infectious diseases such as impetigo and scabies
- droplet-transmitted infectious diseases such as haemophilus influenzae type b, pneumonia, and pertussis
- airborne infectious diseases such as tuberculosis and chicken pox (varicella)
- bloodborne infectious diseases such as human immunodeficiency virus (HIV) and hepatitis B virus (HBV)

. . . .

Nursing Assistant/Nurse Aide Flash Review

CHAIN OF INFECTION

. . . .

ASEPSIS

. . . .

According to the Centers for Disease Control and Prevention, communicable diseases result when the agent leaves its reservoir through a portal of exit, moves by some mode of transmission, and enters through an appropriate portal of entry to infect a susceptible host.

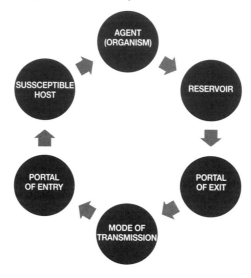

Asepsis is the physical removal of infectious organisms. Techniques include the following:

- Sanitization includes hand washing, cleaning surfaces with soap and water, and providing clean clothing.

- Antisepsis involves killing organisms or stopping them from growing on the skin and other surfaces. Antiseptic chemicals include iodine and alcohol.

- Disinfection is the use of stronger chemicals to kill organisms on contaminated nonliving objects such as bedpans.

- Sterilization uses pressurized steam (autoclave) or prolonged soaking in chemicals to completely remove microbes from objects such as surgical instruments that must be completely germ free.

STANDARD PRECAUTIONS

. . . .

BODY FLUIDS

. . . .

Standard precautions are used for all clients to protect them and others from blood and body fluid pathogens. The following are some standard precautions:

- Hand hygiene includes washing with plain or antibacterial soap and water, and the use of alcohol gel to decontaminate hands.
- Gloves are used for contact with blood and body fluids and excretions.
- Gowns or aprons are used during procedures when the nursing assistant may come into contact with blood or body fluids.
- Masks and protective eyewear are used to protect eyes, mouth, and nose during client activities that may cause spraying or splashing of blood or body fluids.
- Containers are utilized for needles, razors, and other used sharp objects.
- Respiratory hygiene or cough etiquette involves using measures such as covering the nose and mouth when sneezing or coughing to prevent persons with respiratory infections from transmitting their infections to others.

· ·

- blood
- breast milk
- feces
- saliva
- secretions from the nose
- spinal fluid
- sputum
- tears
- urine
- vomit
- wound drainage

· ·

HAND WASHING

. . . .

USING HAND SANITIZER

. . . .

PART
5

Hand washing is the most important way to prevent the spread of infection.

- Assemble equipment (sink with running water, soap, paper towels, waste container).

- Turn on water.

- Thoroughly wet hands and wrists; keep fingertips pointing downward.

- Apply soap to hands.

- Lather and vigorously rub surfaces of wrists, hands, and fingers for at least 15 seconds; keep hands lower than the elbows and the fingertips down.

- Interlace fingers and rub between them.

- Clean fingernails by rubbing fingertips against palm of the opposite hand.

- Rinse all surfaces of wrists, hands, and fingers; keep hands lower than the elbows and the fingertips down.

- Uses clean, dry paper towel(s) to dry all surfaces of hands, wrists, and fingers.

- Dispose of paper towel(s) into waste container.

- Use clean, dry paper towel to turn off faucet.

- Dispose of paper towel(s) into waste container.

- Do not touch inside of sink or waste container at any time.

• •

Hand sanitizer is used as a quick way to perform hand hygiene or when hand washing sinks are not available.

- Locate wall-mounted dispenser.

- Apply the product to the palm of one hand, obtaining enough to cover the skin of both hands (about 1 to 2 mls).

- Rub hands together.

- Rub the product over all surfaces of the hands and fingers until hands are dry (about 30 seconds).

Do not use hand sanitizer when hands are visibly dirty. Hand sanitizer does not remove body fluids or soil from the hands.

• •

PERSONAL PROTECTIVE EQUIPMENT (PPE)

....

GLOVES

....

Personal protective equipment (PPE) includes gloves, gowns, protective eyewear, and masks. They are considered barrier methods of infection control because they physically prevent organisms from contaminating healthcare providers' mucous membranes and skin. All must be removed in a way that prevents the organisms from contaminating the healthcare provider.

. . . .

Gloves provide a barrier between the nursing assistant's hands and body fluids or other contaminants.

Putting on gloves

- Obtain gloves.

- Wash hands.

- Slip on gloves, one at a time.

- Make sure gloves fit comfortably and are not too tight or too loose.

- Inspect gloves for tears.

Taking off gloves

- With both hands still gloved, use the gloved fingers of one glove to grasp the other glove just below the cuff.

- Peel off the glove, inside out.

- Avoid making contact with the inside of the other hand.

- Hold the removed glove with the index finger and thumb of the gloved hand.

- Place the ungloved middle and index finger inside the cuff of the remaining glove.

- Peel off the second glove from the inside, tucking the first glove into the second glove as it is removed.

- Discard gloves in the waste container.

- Wash hands.

. . . .

GOWNS

. . . .

Gowns are barriers to body fluids and other contaminants.

Putting on gown

- Roll up uniform sleeves if they are long.
- Unfold gown.
- Put arms into the sleeves.
- Secure the gown around neck by fastening the ties or closure strips, making sure that uniform is covered.
- Grasp sides of gown and pull back, overlapping the sides to completely cover uniform.
- Secure the gown at the waist by fastening the ties or closure strips.

Taking off gown

- Leave gloves on.
- Undo waist ties or closure strips.
- Undo neck ties or closure strips.
- Grab gown at the shoulder and pull off sleeve, turning sleeve inside out as this is done.
- Repeat with other arm.
- Hold gown away from the body and fold it inside out.
- Dispose of gown in facility-approved container.
- Wash hands.

MASKS

· ·

The proper use of a face mask prevents airborne and droplet organisms from entering the nose and mouth.

Putting on mask

- Place mask over nose and mouth without touching face with hands.
- Tie the top ties behind head.
- Tie the bottom ties behind neck.

Taking off mask

- Wash hands.
- Untie bottom ties.
- Untie top ties.
- Remove mask, holding top ties.
- Dispose of mask in facility-approved container.

· ·

TRANSMISSION-BASED PRECAUTIONS

Transmission-based precautions are used for clients with specific types of infectious diseases. They include contact, droplet, and airborne precautions.

	Contact Precautions	Droplet Precautions	Airborne Precautions
When used	When organisms can be transmitted by direct contact (stool incontinence, draining wounds, uncontrolled secretions, pressure ulcers, or ostomy tubes and/or bags draining body fluids)	When organisms can be transmitted by droplets when coughing	When organisms can be transmitted by droplets that remain in the air
PPE	Gown and gloves when providing care or touching contaminated items	Face mask for close contact with the client; the face mask should be donned upon entering the exam room; if substantial spraying of respiratory fluids is possible, also use protective eyewear	Standard precautions are used for gloves and gowns; N-95 or higher-level masks, if available, when caring for the client; put on mask prior to room entry and remove after exiting room
Client transport	Limit movement and transport	If necessary to move the client, decrease dispersal of droplets by having client wear a mask	Limit transport to essential purposes, and have client wear mask if possible
Client equipment	Linen and waste must be disposed of properly	Clean and disinfect common equipment and items	Equipment must be adequately cleaned before use on another client

Nursing Assistant/Nurse Aide Flash Review

ISOLATION PRECAUTIONS

....

Isolation means that the client is separated from other clients on the unit, and it is usually used when the client has an infectious disease that can be transmitted through the air. When caring for clients in isolation, nursing assistants should:

- Allow for extra time.
- Be efficient to avoid having to leave room during care, thus avoiding unnecessary regowning.
- Be supportive; isolation can create fear, loneliness, and stigma.
- Show clients you are not afraid to care for them.
- Maintain confidentiality.

· ·

Nursing Assistant/Nurse Aide Flash Review

OCCUPATIONAL SAFETY AND HEALTH ADMINISTRATION (OSHA)

. . . .

ENVIRONMENTAL SAFETY HAZARDS

. . . .

PART
5

Congress created the Occupational Safety and Health Administration (OSHA) with the Occupational Safety and Health Act of 1970 to help protect workers from being harmed or killed at their workplace. The purpose of OSHA is to assure safe and healthy working conditions by setting and enforcing standards and by providing training, outreach, education, and assistance. The standards require employers to provide a workplace that is free of known dangers to employees.

. . . .

- bed elevation incorrect
- cluttered paths of travel
- dangerous chemicals
- dim or reduced lighting
- exposure to weather
- frayed cords
- hot liquids or food
- improper shoes or dress
- improper use of equipment
- out-of-reach items
- sharps
- side rails
- slippery surfaces
- smoking
- unlocked wheels
- wet floors

. . . .

Nursing Assistant/Nurse Aide Flash Review

BODY MECHANICS

. . . .

BACK SAFETY

. . . .

FALL PREVENTION

PART
5

Proper body mechanics allows for efficient movement and use of the body. Nursing assistants should follow the ABCs of body mechanics:

- Alignment is good posture with the back in a neutral position and the curve of the lower back intact.

- Balance is the even distribution of body weight to create stability by maintaining the person's center of gravity close to the base of support.

- Coordinated body movement involves using one's body weight for movement.

· ·

To prevent back and other injury, the nursing assistant should use proper body mechanics:

- Assess the situation and ask for assistance if you think you will be unable to move the person or object alone.

- Position your body close to the person or object to be lifted or moved.

- Use correct posture and keep body aligned (back straight, knees bent).

- Use wide base of support with your feet aligned in front of your work and apart at shoulder width.

- Do not use back and arms for lifting.

- Turn or pivot your feet; do not twist your body.

- Use smooth movements and avoid sudden jerky motions.

- Use both hands when lifting.

· ·

Healthcare providers are at risk for falls. Factors that increase risk include wet floors, being in a hurry, objects in the walking path, and poor lighting. To help prevent falls, nursing assistants can be aware of their surroundings, contact the appropriate department to clean up spills, position objects so they are not in the way of walking, and utilize adequate lighting.

CHEMICAL INJURY PREVENTION

. . . .

ELECTRICAL SHOCK PREVENTION

. . . .

FIRE PREVENTION

PART 5

Many chemicals, including cleaning solutions and chemotherapeutic medications, can cause harm if inhaled, ingested, or absorbed through the skin. Other chemicals can become harmful when mixed with other products. OSHA requires facilities to educate workers about the chemicals in their workplace. One way to do this is through the use of material safety data sheets (MSDSs) that chemical substance manufactures are required to supply. MSDSs provide information that includes chemical makeup of the substance, the exposure types that can be dangerous, what to do if exposed, and how to manage spills. Nursing assistants are responsible for the safe handling of the chemicals that they use in their facilities.

· ·

Healthcare facilities are filled with electrical equipment. Most equipment should be grounded by either a three-pronged plug or a ground-fault breaker. To prevent electrical shock, nursing assistants should report defective equipment, including those that have frayed wires and loose plugs, and should be aware of the potential hazards of using electrical equipment near water.

· ·

Fires require three elements: heat, fuel, and oxygen. Heat can come from smoking materials, candles, furnaces, and electrical sparks; fuel can be clothing, bedding, paper, and the facility building; oxygen is in room air and in oxygen tanks. To help prevent fires, nursing assistants can:

- Know the facility's fire safety policies.

- Know the facility's exits.

- Keep combustible substances away from oxygen sources.

- Make sure electrical equipment is in working order.

- Avoid using flammable substances near heat sources.

- If smoking is permitted in the facility:
  - Disallow clients to smoke in bed.
  - Supervise clients when smoking.
  - Keep smoking materials safely away from children and confused clients.

Nursing Assistant/Nurse Aide Flash Review

FIRE EMERGENCY RESPONSE

. . . .

FIRE EXTINGUISHERS

. . . .

DISASTER PREPAREDNESS

PART
5

Fires can occur, even when safety precautions are used. Should a fire occur, follow the RACE response plan:

- **R**emove clients in immediate danger to a place of safety.
- **A**ctivate the alarm and follow the facility's policy for reporting a fire.
- **C**onfine the fire by closing doors and windows.
- **E**xtinguish the fire if it is small or **E**vacuate the building if it is too large for a fire extinguisher.

• •

Not all fires are the same, so fires are classified by type:

- Class A: fires with common materials such as trash, wood, paper
- Class B: fires with flammable or combustible petroleum-based liquids
- Class C: fires that involve electrical equipment

A type ABC fire extinguisher can be used for all types of fires. When using a fire extinguisher, use the PASS system:

- **P**ull the safety pin.
- **A**im at the base of the fire.
- **S**queeze the trigger.
- **S**weep the spray from side to side.

• •

Disasters are sudden events such as hurricanes, blizzards, and terrorist attacks, which can result in numerous casualities and significant property damage. Nursing assistants are required to know their facility's disaster plan, which is usually reviewed annually and practiced in drills.

WORKPLACE VIOLENCE

OSHA notes that workplace violence is violence or the threat of violence against workers that may occur at or outside the workplace. It can range from verbal abuse to physical assaults and homicide, and is one of the leading causes of job-related deaths. According to the OSHA Guidelines for Preventing Workplace Violence for Health Care and Social Service Workers, increased risk of work-related assaults comes from several factors, including:

- the prevalence of handguns and other weapons among patients, their families, or friends
- the increasing use of hospitals by police and the criminal justice system for criminal holds and the care of acutely disturbed, violent individuals
- the increasing number of acute and chronic mentally ill patients being released from hospitals without follow-up care (these patients have the right to refuse medicine and can no longer be hospitalized involuntarily unless they pose an immediate threat to themselves or others)
- the availability of drugs or money at hospitals, clinics, and pharmacies, making them likely robbery targets
- factors such as the unrestricted movement of the public in clinics and hospitals and long waits in emergency or clinic areas that lead to client frustration over an inability to obtain needed services promptly
- the increasing presence of gang members, drug or alcohol abusers, trauma patients, or distraught family members
- low staffing levels during times of increased activity such as mealtimes, visiting times, and when staff is transporting patients
- isolated work with clients during examinations or treatment
- solo work, often in remote locations with no backup or way to get assistance, such as communication devices or alarm systems (this is particularly true in high-crime settings)
- lack of staff training in recognizing and managing escalating hostile and assaultive behavior
- poorly lit parking areas

Healthcare workers, therefore, receive training to protect themselves from workplace violence.

• •

Nursing Assistant/Nurse Aide Flash Review

FOLLOWING PROCEDURES

Nursing assistants can minimize injury to self and others by following procedures, including pre- and postprocedure protocols:

- Preprocedure protocols
    - Obtain necessary supplies.
    - Wash hands and apply gloves (when required).
    - Identify self and position to the client and greet the person.
    - Explain the procedure.
    - Provide privacy.
    - Follow safety precautions.

- Postprocedure protocols
    - Make sure the client is comfortable.
    - Lower the bed and raise the side rail (if needed for that client).
    - Leave the call bell within the client's reach.
    - Wash hands.
    - Report and document as required.

. . . .

EMERGENCIES

. . . .

EMERGENCY MEDICAL SERVICES

. . . .

PART 5

RESPONDING TO AN EMERGENCY

Emergencies are events that require immediate action.

. . . .

Emergency medical technicians (EMTs) answer emergency calls, drive ambulances, and give basic medical care. Some EMTs are paramedics and have training to do medical procedures on-site. Emergency medical services are usually accessed when a person dials 911. After dialing 911 (or another appropriate emergency number), the caller will be expected to provide:

- the nature of the emergency

- the phone number the caller is calling from

- the number of people needing assistance

- what is being done for the person(s) in need of emergency assistance

. . . .

The nursing assistant's responsibilities in an emergency are:

- recognizing that an emergency exists

- making the decision to act

- checking for the client's level of consciousness

- activating the emergency response system

- providing appropriate care until EMTs or other appropriate personnel arrive

- reporting and documenting this care

RESPONDING TO FAINTING

. . . .

RESPONDING TO SEIZURES

. . . .

Fainting, also called syncope or passing out, is a brief and sudden loss of consciousness that results from a loss of blood flow to the brain. Fainting can happen at any age and may be caused by a number of problems, including stress, pain, fatigue, heat, dehydration, pregnancy, diabetes, anemia, and heart disease. When responding to a client who has fainted:

- Call for assistance as needed.

- Get the client into a supine position and elevate the feet to increase blood circulation to the brain.

- Make sure the client has a strong pulse and is breathing easily.

- Apply a cool cloth to the client's head.

- Report and document.

Seizures (convulsions) are partial or generalized episodes that result from abnormal brain activity. Seizures vary. Generalized seizures range from absence (petit mal) seizures, where a person may just stop and stare, to tonic-clonic (grand mal) seizures, where the person may lose consciousness and alternate between violent jerking and rigidity. Partial seizures include complex seizures, where the person exhibits involuntary coordinated movements such as lip smacking, and simple motor seizures, where the person has jerking or muscle rigidity in one area of the body. Seizures can last from seconds to minutes, but the rare status epilepticus can last for hours. When responding to a client who is having a significant seizure:

- Call for assistance.

- Keep the person safe.

- If the person is sitting or standing when the seizure starts, help him or her to the floor.

- Move away furniture or objects that may cause harm.

- Protect the person's head by placing a pillow or folded towel under it.

- Do not place anything in the person's mouth.

- Once the seizure is over, place the person in the recovery position by turning him or her on the side to allow secretions to flow from the mouth.

- Report and document.

Nursing Assistant/Nurse Aide Flash Review

RESPONDING TO BURNS

. . . .

PART 5

Burns are injuries to the skin and other tissue caused by heat or fire (thermal burns), electricity (electrical burns), chemicals (chemical burns), or radiation (radiation burns, such as sunburn).

Burns are classified by their depth:

- superficial partial thickness (first degree): outer layer damaged; painful and red
- partial thickness (second degree): epidermis and upper layer of dermis damaged; red, blisters, painful, minimal scarring
- full thickness (third degree): epidermis and dermis damaged, may involve underlying tissue, nerve endings usually destroyed; skin dark red to black to white, usually no pain

When responding to a client who is burned:

Superficial

- Flush area with cold water.
- Cover area with a sterile dressing.

Partial or full thickness

- Remove the heat source and stop the burning process.
- Call for assistance.
- Keep airway open.
- Cover the area with a sterile dressing.
- Do not remove stuck clothing.
- Observe for signs of shock.

RESPONDING TO POISONING

Poisons are substances that act as toxins in the body. A number of sub-stances, including medications and plants, can act as poisons, and persons can be poisoned by inhaling, ingesting, injecting, or absorbing a poison-ous substance. When responding to a client who has been poisoned:

- Check the mouth for signs of burns and significant odors.
- Look for the container that may contain the poison.
- Call Poison Control (1-800-222-1222).
- Follow directions from Poison Control.
- Call for emergency assistance.
- Keep person warm.
- Follow other emergency procedures as needed.

. . . .

Nursing Assistant/Nurse Aide Flash Review

RESPONDING TO SHOCK

Shock is a life-threatening condition that occurs when the cardiovascular system does not pump enough oxygenated blood to the body. There are several different types of shock:

- hemorrhagic from blood loss
- respiratory from impaired breathing that reduces the amount of oxygen in the blood
- neurogenic from loss of nervous system control
- psychogenic from a sudden widening of the blood vessels that decreases blood flow to the brain
- cardiogenic from inadequate cardiac functioning
- septic from infection that may dilate the blood vessels or create clots
- metabolic from fluid loss or body chemical changes
- anaphylactic from severe allergy

Symptoms of shock include anxiety, thirst, dull appearance to the eyes, dilated pupils, cold and clammy skin, rapid and weak pulse, nausea, vomiting, and collapse. Immediate treatment is needed to prevent organ damage and death. When responding to a client who is in shock or is going into shock:

- Call for assistance.
- Stay with the person.
- Do not let the person move unnecessarily, eat, drink, or smoke.
- Ensure that the person is breathing, and check pulse and level of consciousness.
- Get the person into a supine position and elevate the feet.
- Loosen tight clothing.
- Cover the person with a blanket.
- Report and document.

Nursing Assistant/Nurse Aide Flash Review

RESPONDING TO HEMORRHAGE

. . . .

RESPONDING TO STROKE

PART 5

. . . .

Hemorrhage is an unexpected and extreme loss of blood that is usually due to trauma or problems with blood clotting. Symptoms include decreased blood pressure, increased pulse, shallow and rapid respirations, cold and moist skin, weakness, restlessness, pallor, and thirst. When responding to a client who is hemorrhaging:

- Call for assistance.

- If the bleeding is external, apply direct pressure while following standard precautions.

- Apply a dressing and monitor it for bleeding.

- If possible, elevate the bleeding area.

- Cover person with a blanket.

- If bleeding is from an artery (spurting, bright red blood), apply pressure to a pressure point (site where the artery lies near the surface of the body and over a bone).

- Use a tourniquet only as a last resort.

. . . .

A cerebral vascular accident (CVA), also known as a stroke or brain attack, happens when the blood flow is blocked or interrupted to part of the brain. Most strokes are caused by either a clot forming (thrombotic stroke) in one of the brain arteries or a clot forming elsewhere (usually the heart), breaking off, and traveling to the brain. Some strokes result from bleeding when a blood vessel in the brain leaks or ruptures; this can be caused by uncontrolled high blood pressure, an aneurysm (weak spot in a blood vessel), trauma, anticoagulant medication, or a bleeding disorder such as hemophilia. Symptoms of a stroke are sudden severe headache, for no reason, dizziness, loss of balance or coordination, confusion, slurred or garbled speech or difficulty understanding others, sudden blindness in one or both eyes or double vision, drooping of one side of the mouth, as well as sudden weakness, numbness, or paralysis in the face, arm, or leg, usually on one side of the body. Symptoms vary according to the location of the stroke in the brain. When responding to a client who is having a stroke:

- Call for assistance, as early treatment can minimize the damage from strokes.

- Keep the person lying down.

- Assess breathing and heart rate.

. . . .

RESPONDING TO HEART ATTACK

. . . .

CARDIOPULMONARY RESUSCITATION (CPR)

. . . .

PART
5

Myocardial infarction (MI) is also called a heart attack. One or more of the coronary arteries blocks completely. This prevents blood from reaching parts of the heart muscle and oxygenating them. The muscle areas then die (infarct). Severity depends on the location and the extent of the damage. Signs of a heart attack include pressure, tightness, pain, or a squeezing or aching sensation in the chest or arms that may spread to the neck, jaw, or back; shortness of breath; a feeling of fullness, nausea, indigestion, heartburn, or abdominal pain; sweating or a cold sweat; feeling of anxiety or an impending sense of doom; fatigue; and lightheadedness or dizziness. When responding to a client who is having a heart attack:

- Call for assistance. Early detection and treatment increase a person's chance of survival.

- Have the person lie down.

- Raise the person's head to improve breathing.

- Begin cardiopulmonary resuscitation (CPR) if the person stops breathing or loses his or her pulse.

. . . .

Cardiopulmonary resuscitation (CPR) is an emergency lifesaving procedure performed when someone's breathing or heartbeat stops, usually after a heart attack, electrical shock, or drowning. CPR combines rescue breathing that provides oxygen to the person's lungs, along with chest compressions that keep oxygen-rich blood flowing until the person's heartbeat and breathing can be restored. CPR techniques vary depending on the age or size of the patient; however, techniques now emphasize compression over rescue breathing, reversing long-standing practice. Time is critical when a person stops breathing because permanent brain damage begins after only four minutes without oxygen, and death can occur as soon as four to six minutes later.

. . . .

ADULT CPR

. . . .

CHILD (1 TO 8 YEARS OLD) CPR

. . . .

The following is based on the American Heart Association instructions:

1. Check for responsiveness.

2. Call 911 if there is no response.

3. Carefully place the person on his or her back.

4. Assess the person's pulse for no more than 10 seconds.

5. Perform chest compressions: Give 30 chest compressions by placing the heel of one hand on the middle of the person's chest and placing the heel of the other hand on top of the first hand. Compress at a rate of at least 100 compressions per minute.

6. Open the airway.

7. Look, listen, and feel for breathing.

8. If the person is not breathing or has trouble breathing: Give two rescue breaths, each taking one second to make the chest rise.

9. Continue CPR (30 chest compressions followed by two breaths, then repeat) until the person recovers or help arrives.

10. If an adult automated external defibrillator (AED) is available, use it as soon as possible.

· ·

The following is based on the American Heart Association instructions:

1. Check for alertness.

2. If there is no response, shout for help. Do not leave the child alone until CPR has been done for about two minutes.

3. Carefully place the child on his or her back.

4. Perform chest compressions at a rate of at least 100 compressions per minute. Give 30 fast chest compressions by placing the heel of one hand on the breast-bone, just below the nipples.

5. Open the airway.

6. Look, listen, and feel for breathing.

7. If the child is not breathing: Give two rescue breaths, each taking one second to make the chest rise.

8. Continue CPR (30 chest compressions followed by two breaths, then repeat).

9. After about two minutes of CPR, if the child still does not have normal breathing, coughing, or movement, call 911. If a child AED is available, use it now.

10. Repeat rescue breathing and chest compressions until the child recovers or help arrives.

· ·

Nursing Assistant/Nurse Aide Flash Review

INFANT CPR

. . . .

CHOKING

. . . .

PART
5

The following is based on the American Heart Association instructions:

1. Check for alertness.

2. If there is no response, shout for help. Do not leave the infant alone until CPR has been done for about two minutes.

3. Carefully place the infant on his or her back.

4. Perform chest compressions at a rate of at least 100 compressions per minute. Give 30 fast chest compressions by placing two fingers on the breastbone, just below the nipples.

5. Open the airway.

6. Look, listen, and feel for breathing.

7. If the infant is not breathing: Give two rescue breaths, each taking one second to make the chest rise.

8. Continue CPR (30 chest compressions followed by two breaths, then repeat) for about two minutes.

9. After about two minutes of CPR, if the infant still does not have normal breathing, coughing, or movement, call 911.

10. Repeat rescue breathing and chest compressions until the infant recovers or help arrives.

. . . .

Choking results in blockage of the airway. The person cannot speak or breathe and can develop cardiac arrest from the lack of oxygen. The universal sign of choking is the person clutching the throat with the hands.

. . . .

RESPONDING TO CHOKING IN PERSONS 1 YEAR OF AGE AND OLDER

PART
5

The American Red Cross recommends a "five-and-five" approach for choking:

- Confirm obstruction.

- Deliver five back blows between the person's shoulder blades with the heel of the hand.

- Perform five abdominal thrusts (also known as the Heimlich maneuver).

- Alternate between five blows and five thrusts until the blockage is dislodged.

- If the person loses consciousness, lower him or her to the floor and continue care.

- Determine unresponsiveness by asking the person if he or she is okay.

- If there is no response, call 911.

- Open the airway and check for air movement.

- Attempt to ventilate the victim.

- If unsuccessful, reposition the head and try again.

- If still unsuccessful, straddle the victim, position one hand on top of the other, and provide three to five upward thrusts between the navel and the sternum.

- If the foreign body is visible in the person's mouth, remove it.

- If it is not visible, repeat thrusts until it dislodges.

- Begin CPR if needed.

(The American Heart Association does not recommend back blows. Both approaches are acceptable.)

. . . .

RESPONDING TO CHOKING IN INFANTS LESS THAN 1 YEAR

. . . .

PART 5

Confirm obstruction.

- Hold infant on arm face down and give five back blows.
- Reposition infant face up on other arm and give five chest thrusts.
- Inspect the mouth and remove any visible foreign body.
- Repeat sequence of five back blows and five chest thrusts until object is expelled.
- Begin CPR if needed.

PURPOSE OF VITAL SIGNS

. . . .

FACTORS THAT AFFECT VITAL SIGNS

. . . .

TEMPERATURE: BASICS

PART
5

Vital signs monitor the essential functioning of body organs. They show the person's state of health and well-being, and they often act as the first sign that something is wrong. Traditional vital signs are temperature, pulse, respirations, and blood pressure. Pain is also now considered a vital sign. Vital signs are obtained:

- upon admission

- as part of the plan of care

- when there is an unusual situation, such as an incident

- when a person complains of unusual symptoms or pain

- to measure response to treatment

· ·

Factors that affect vital signs include age, exercise, environmental temperature, medications, and emotions.

· ·

Temperature (i.e., the amount of body heat) is measured with a thermometer (digital, battery-operated electronic, tympanic, temporal, oral plastic, and the forehead thermometer strip). The mouth (oral), ear (tympanic), forehead (temporal), armpit (axillary), and rectum (rectal) are the most common sites for assessing temperature, and the nursing assistant should record the method used:

- oral = O

- tympanic = T

- temporal = TA

- axillary = A

- rectal = R

TEMPERATURE: CHARACTERISTICS

. . . .

TEMPERATURE: PROCEDURE FOR ORAL TEMPERATURE WITH AN ELECTRONIC THERMOMETER

. . . .

Temperature readings are recorded in either degrees Fahrenheit (°F) or degrees Celsius (°C), depending on facility preference. Normal body temperature is 98.6°F or 37°C. To convert from one type to the other:

- $C = \frac{5}{9} (F - 32)$
- $F = (\frac{9}{5} C) + 32$

Temperature fluctuates with the body's circadian rhythm, with the temperature being elevated between 5 P.M. and 7 P.M. Normal monthly fluctuations in women occur with the menstrual cycle.

· ·

To take an oral temperature with an electronic thermometer:

- Gather equipment.
- Explain procedure to client.
- Perform hand hygiene and put on gloves.
- Place disposable protective sheath over probe.
- Place tip of thermometer under the client's tongue along the gum line.
- Instruct client to keep mouth closed.
- Read measurement on digital display of electronic thermometer when it signals and displays a constant temperature.
- Push ejection button to discard disposable sheath into receptacle.
- Remove gloves and perform hand hygiene.
- Record reading according to institution policies and report abnormal temperatures.

· ·

Nursing Assistant/Nurse Aide Flash Review

TEMPERATURE: PROCEDURE FOR TYMPANIC TEMPERATURE

. . . .

To take a tympanic temperature:

- Gather equipment.

- Explain procedure to client.

- Perform hand hygiene.

- Remove probe from container, and attach it to the tympanic thermometer unit.

- Turn client's head to one side:
    - For an adult, pull pinna upward and back.
    - For a child, pull pinna down and back.

- Gently insert probe with firm pressure into ear canal.

- Read measurement on digital display of electronic thermometer when it signals and displays a constant temperature.

- Remove probe cover and discard disposable sheath into receptacle.

- Perform hand hygiene.

- Record reading according to institution policies and report abnormal temperatures.

. . . .

TEMPERATURE: PROCEDURE FOR AXILLARY TEMPERATURE

. . . .

PART
5

To take an axillary temperature:

- Gather equipment.

- Explain procedure to client.

- Perform hand hygiene.

- Provide for privacy.

- Remove probe from container, and attach it to the thermometer unit.

- Make sure axillary skin is dry; if not, pat dry.

- Place probe into center of axilla. Fold the client's upper arm straight down, and place arm across the client's chest.

- Read measurement on digital display of electronic thermometer when it signals and displays a constant temperature.

- Remove probe cover and discard disposable sheath into receptacle.

- Perform hand hygiene.

- Record reading according to institution policies and report abnormal temperatures.

TEMPERATURE: PROCEDURE FOR RECTAL TEMPERATURE

. . . .

To take a rectal temperature:

- Gather equipment.

- Explain procedure to client.

- Perform hand hygiene.

- Provide for privacy.

- Remove probe from container, and attach it to the thermometer unit.

- Place client in the Sims' position with upper knee flexed, making sure to use a sheet to cover client and expose only the anal area.

- Lubricate tip of rectal (red cap) probe.

- Grasp top of the probe's stem with dominant hand, and separate buttocks to expose the anus with the other hand.

- Instruct the client to take a deep breath.

- Insert the probe gently into anus about $\frac{1}{2}$ inch. Do not force insertion if resistance is felt.

- Read measurement on digital display of electronic thermometer when it signals and displays a constant temperature.

- Remove probe cover and discard disposable sheath into receptacle.

- Remove gloves and perform hand hygiene.

- Record reading according to institution policies and report abnormal temperatures.

. . . .

Nursing Assistant/Nurse Aide Flash Review

PULSE: BASICS

....

PULSE: CHARACTERISTICS

....

PART
5

The pulse is a basic measure of cardiovascular functioning. It shows how fast the heart is beating. The pulse can be measured at several pulse points (where an artery can easily be felt because it is close to the body's surface): carotid, radial, brachial, femoral, popliteal, posterior tibial, and dorsalis pedis. The radial pulse, which is located near the base of the thumb on the palm side of the wrist, is the most common choice to assess the pulse. The pulse may also be assessed at the apex of the heart (the apical pulse), which is located just below the left breast and assessed using a stethoscope. The radial and apical pulse rates should be the same.

· ·

When assessing and recording the pulse, nursing assistants will note the rate, rhythm, and force of the heartbeat:

- Rate is the number of beats per minute.
    - Normal adult rate is 60 to 80 beats per minute.
    - Normal infant rate is 80 to 160 beats per minute.
    - Normal child rate is 80 to 115 beats per minute.
    - Normal older adult rate is 60 to 70 beats per minute.
    - Bradycardia is a slow heart rate (under 60 for adults).
    - Tachycardia is a fast heart rate (over 100 for adults).

- Rhythm is the regularity of the heartbeats
    - Regular rhythm means that the length of time between beats is consistent.
    - Irregular rhythm means that the length of time between beats is inconsistent.

- Force is the strength of the heartbeats.
    - Weak pulse is difficult to feel.
    - Strong pulse is easy to feel.

· ·

Nursing Assistant/Nurse Aide Flash Review

PULSE: PROCEDURE FOR RADIAL PULSE

. . . .

PULSE: PROCEDURE FOR APICAL PULSE

. . . .

Explain procedure to client.

- Perform hand hygiene.
- Bend client's elbow and place the lower part of the arm across the chest.
- Support client's wrist by holding outer aspect with thumb.
- Place index and middle fingers over the radial artery, and apply light but firm pressure until pulse is palpated.
- Identify pulse rhythm and strength.
- Determine pulse rate using a watch with a second hand:
  - If the rhythm is regular, count the beats for 30 seconds and multiply by 2.
  - If the rhythm is irregular, count the beats for a full minute.
- Perform hand hygiene.
- Record reading according to institution policies and report abnormal pulses. Pulse rate should be within plus or minus four beats of nurse's reading.

. . . .

Explain procedure to client.

- Perform hand hygiene.
- Clean earpieces and diaphragm of stethoscope with an alcohol swab.
- Locate apex of heart.
- Instruct client to remain silent and breathe normally through the nose.
- Put earpiece of the stethoscope in ears and warm the diaphragm in the palm of the hand for 5 to 10 seconds.
- Uncover the left side of the client's chest, without overexposing the client.
- Place diaphragm of stethoscope at the fifth intercostal space to the left of the sternum.
- Listen to the heartbeats and note their rhythm and strength.
- Count the heartbeats for a full minute (each lub-dub [the two normal heart sounds] equals one beat)
- Perform hand hygiene.
- Record reading according to institution policies and report abnormal pulse rates.

. . . .

RESPIRATION: BASICS

. . . .

RESPIRATION: CHARACTERISTICS

. . . .

Respiration is the process of inspiration/inhaling (breathing in, causing the chest to expand) and expiration/exhaling (breathing out, causing the chest to contract). Each respiratory cycle consists of one inhalation and one exhalation, or one breath.

Respiratory rate varies by age:

- Less than 1 month: 30 to 60 breaths per minute

- 1 to 6 months: 30 to 50 breaths per minute

- 6 to 12 months: 24 to 46 breaths per minute

- 1 to 4 years: 20 to 30 breaths per minute

- 4 to 6 years: 20 to 25 breaths per minute

- 6 to 12 years: 16 to 20 breaths per minute

- Greater than 12 years and adult: 12 to 16 breaths per minute

- Tachypnea means respiratory rate is too rapid.

- Bradypnea means respiratory rate is too slow.

The quality of respiration is as important as the rate:

- Apnea means the absence of breathing.

- Dyspnea means labored respirations.

- Abdominal respiration means that respirations are being assisted primarily with the abdominal muscles.

- Shallow respirations means the person is breathing with only the upper part of the lungs.

- Hyperpnea is increased rate and depth of respiration.

Nursing Assistant/Nurse Aide Flash Review

RESPIRATIONS: PROCEDURE

. . . .

BLOOD PRESSURE: BASICS

. . . .

PART
5

Explain procedure to client.

- Perform hand hygiene.

- After assessing the radial pulse, leave finger on the radial artery and observe respirations. Do not inform the client about assessing respirations because this can cause the person to change his or her breathing pattern.

- Observe both the rise and the fall of the client's chest and count this as one breath.

- Monitor respiratory depth and rhythm.

- If respirations are regular, count them for 30 seconds and multiply by 2. If they are irregular, count them for a full minute.

- Perform hand hygiene.

- Record reading according to institution policies and report abnormal respirations. Respiration rate must be within plus or minus two breaths of nurse's reading.

• •

The blood pressure is a measurement of the force of blood through the arteries as pumped by the heart. Pressure is highest when the heart contracts; this is the systolic pressure. Pressure is lowest when the heart relaxes; this is the diastolic pressure. Both are measured when taking a client's blood pressure, usually using a digital or aneroid (dial) sphygmomanometer.

• •

BLOOD PRESSURE: CHARACTERISTICS

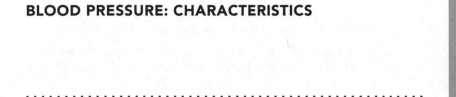

BLOOD PRESSURE: PROCEDURE

PART 5

In healthy adults, the normal systolic pressure is 120mm Hg, and the normal diastolic pressure is 80mm Hg. This is documented as 120/80. Blood pressure can be affected by stress, anger, or fear, as well as medications, illicit substances, neurological or cardiac disorders, hemorrhage, shock, burns, and preeclampsia.

- Hypotension, or low blood pressure, exists when the systolic pressure is less than 90mm Hg and/or the diastolic pressure is less than 60mm Hg.

- Hypertension, or high blood pressure, exists when the systolic pressure is above 140mm Hg and/or the diastolic pressure is above 90mm Hg.

. . . .

Gather appropriate equipment, including a stethoscope and sphygmomanometer, making sure to choose the appropriate cuff size. Clean earpieces and diaphragm of stethoscope with alcohol wipes.

- Explain procedure to client.

- Perform hand hygiene.

- Position the client's arm with palm up and elbow at the level of the heart.

- Wrap cuff evenly around arm, keeping the cuff bladder over the brachial artery, with bottom of cuff positioned within an inch above the antecubital area.

- Locate the brachial artery with fingertips.

- Position diaphragm of stethoscope over brachial artery.

- Place stethoscope earpieces in ears.

- Inflate cuff quickly to 30mm Hg higher than when pulse was last felt.

- Control deflation of cuff and listen for blood pressure sounds.

- The first clear sound is the systolic pressure.

- The diastolic pressure is noted right when sound is no longer heard.

- Fully deflate cuff and remove it from the client's arm.

- Clean earpieces and diaphragm of stethoscope with alcohol wipes again.

- Perform hand hygiene.

- Record reading according to institution policies and report abnormal blood pressures. Both systolic and diastolic pressures should be within plus or minus 8mm of nurse's reading.

. . . .

Nursing Assistant/Nurse Aide Flash Review

PAIN: BASICS

· ·

PAIN: MEASUREMENT

· ·

WEIGHT AND HEIGHT: BASICS

PART 5

Pain is considered the fifth vital sign. Pain has many causes, including trauma, cancer, infection, inflammation, wounds, and emotional distress. Culture plays a key role in pain, and some cultures may be stoic and not complain of pain. It is important to notice and report clients' pain so that it can be managed to make the client more comfortable.

. . . .

Nursing assistants play a key role in noticing that clients may be in pain. There are several scales used to allow clients to rate their pain. One is the numerical scale where clients rate their pain from 0 to 10, with 0 being no pain and 10 being the worst possible pain. Another example is the Wong-Baker FACES® Pain Rating Scale that uses faces to help clients, especially children, rate the severity of their pain.

. . . .

Weight and height are measured to assess clients' nutritional level. Weight is also used to calculate medication dosages and assess the progress of certain diseases and dehydration. Clients should be weighed at the same time each day, and devices such as casts can falsely affect the reading. Weight is measured in either pounds or kilograms, depending on the facility's policy. Height is measured in feet and/or inches or in centimeters, depending on the facility's policy.

Nursing Assistant/Nurse Aide Flash Review

WEIGHT MEASUREMENT OF AMBULATORY CLIENT

- Explain procedure.
- Wash hands.
- Make sure client wears shoes before walking onto scale.
- Set scale to zero.
- Stand next to client as he or she steps onto scale, and assist client, if needed, onto center of the scale.
- Determine the client's weight.
- Stand next to client as he or she steps off scale, and assist client if needed.
- Record weight. Weight should be within plus or minus 2 pounds of nurse's reading or within plus or minus 0.9 kg of nurse's reading.

. . . .

Nursing Assistant/Nurse Aide Flash Review

WEIGHT USING BED SCALE

- Explain procedure to client.
- Perform hand hygiene.
- Set the bed level.
- Ensure that client is lying flat in bed.
- Balance the bed scale.
- Assist client in rolling on side, facing away from the nursing assistant.
- Slide bed scale sling lengthwise next to client, including the client's head.
- Assist client in rolling to the opposite side, facing the nursing assistant.
- Pull the bed scale sling under the client and assist client with rolling on back onto the sling.
- Center the bed scale over the bed and carefully lower and attach the arms to the sling. Lock scale in place.
- Have client keep arms at side during the procedure to prevent injury.
- Lock the hydraulic mechanism and pump bed scale handle to raise client a few inches off the bed.
- Make sure nothing (catheters, IVs, etc.) is pulling on the sling and affecting the weight measurement.
- Push button and read weight.
- Release the hydraulic mechanism and lower client back onto the bed. Disconnect the sling from the arms.
- Release the locks and move the scale away from the bed.
- Assist client in rolling off the sling, and remove sling from bed.
- Perform hand hygiene.
- Record reading according to institution policies and report abnormal weights.

· ·

HEIGHT MEASUREMENT OF CLIENT IN BED

. . . .

- Explain procedure to client.
- Perform hand hygiene.
- With client in a supine position, have client stretch as much as possible.
- Place tape measure on the bed next to the client and extend it from the top of the head to the bottom of the feet.
- Measure the distance.
- Perform hand hygiene.
- Record reading according to institution policies and report abnormal heights.

Nursing Assistant/Nurse Aide Flash Review

DAILY CARE

. . . .

Daily care is provided to all clients in an unhurried manner and as permissible for the client's condition:

- Morning care before breakfast: assist with elimination needs; wash client's hands and face; assist with oral hygiene; provide fresh water if permissible; raise head and reposition if permissible; clean over-bed table.

- Morning care after breakfast: assist with elimination needs; assist with oral hygiene and bathing; change client's gown/clothing; shave if permissible; reposition as permitted; tidy the room and make the bed.

- Afternoon care after lunch: assist with elimination needs; wash client's hands and face; assist with oral hygiene; provide fresh water if permissible; change clothing as needed; reposition if permissible; tidy the area.

- Evening care before bedtime: assist with elimination needs; wash client's hands and face; assist with oral hygiene; provide back rub if desired and permissible; change draw sheet if needed; offer an extra blanket; provide fresh water if permissible; quiet and darken room for sleep.

Nursing Assistant/Nurse Aide Flash Review

ORAL CARE: TEETH

· ·

Oral hygiene is an important part of daily personal care. It helps remove bad tastes from medications and illness, as well as tongue coatings that can interfere with taste. To provide oral care for clients, nursing assistants will:

- Wash hands and put on gloves.

- Explain the procedure to the client.

- Place the client in a sitting position at a 45-degree angle to prevent choking, if allowed

- Place towel or protective cover over the client's clothing and top sheet to keep them clean and dry.

- Remove dentures if present.

- If the client needs assistance, wet the toothbrush with water and put toothpaste on it.

- Carefully brush all surfaces of the teeth.

- Have the client rinse mouth with water or mouthwash.

- Floss between the teeth with dental floss, but wear a face mask due to the potential for gum bleeding and splashing.

- Remove gloves and wash hands.

- If any of the following are noticed during oral care, report and document them: pain, sores, redness, coating of the tongue or cheeks, broken teeth or dentures, and bad breath.

· ·

ORAL CARE: DENTURES

PART
5

Dentures are full or partial sets of false teeth. They are expensive and require careful handling. To care for dentures:

- Wash hands and put on gloves.

- Have client remove dentures or remove dentures for him or her.

- Line sink with a paper towel or water to help avoid denture breakage if dropped.

- Use cool or room-temperature water, not hot water, which can damage dentures.

- Rinse the dentures.

- Carefully brush dentures using a toothbrush and denture cleanser or toothpaste while holding them safely and firmly in the hand.

- Rinse dentures under the running water.

- Place the dentures in a denture cup or emesis basin with cool water or mouthwash, and put them back in the client's mouth after mouth care.

- If the client removes the dentures at night, they should be cleaned and put in the denture cup with water, mouthwash, or a denture cleaning tablet until the morning. Cup should be labeled with client's name and room number and kept in a safe place to prevent damage or accidental disposal into the trash.

- Remove gloves and wash hands when finished.

. . . .

ORAL CARE: UNCONSCIOUS PERSON

· ·

- Gather equipment.

- Wash hands and put on gloves.

- Talk to client and explain what is being done throughout the procedure since an unconscious client may be able to hear.

- Stand at the side of the bed and turn client's head toward the nursing assistant.

- Place towel and emesis basin under client's chin.

- Open client's mouth by placing gentle pressure to chin—do not put fingers in client's mouth.

- Wipe client's mouth with mouth care swabs.

- Drop used swabs in basin and dry client's mouth with towel.

- Place lubricant on client's lips, using an applicator.

- Remove gloves and wash hands.

BATHING CLIENTS

There are four types of baths: showers for clients who are strong enough to get out of bed, tub baths for clients who need them for therapeutic reasons, partial baths for clients who can do most of their own bathing but who need help with hard-to-reach areas, and complete baths for clients who are too ill or weak to do their own care. To perform a complete bed bath, the nursing assistant should:

- Gather equipment.
- Wash hands and put on gloves.
- Provide privacy and raise bed to a comfortable working level.
- Place client in supine position near the side of the bed nearest the nursing assistant.
- Cover top sheet with a large towel and ask client to hold towel in place. If the client is unable, tuck sheet under client's shoulders.
- Remove top sheet and place in laundry basket at bedside.
- Remove client's gown.
- Fill bath basin two-thirds full of warm water.
- Place a towel across the client's chest.
- Wet washcloth, squeeze out excess water, and make a washcloth mitt.
- Wash eyes first, starting at inner corner and working out. Use different area of washcloth for each eye. Do not use soap near the eyes.
- Wash, rinse, and dry face, ears, nose, and mouth area, using soap only if requested by client.
- Wash, rinse, and dry neck.
- Expose farther arm; place towel under arm up to axilla. Wash and rinse far shoulder, axilla, arm, and hand. If the client is able, place a basin of water on the bed, immerse client's hand in water, and wash.
- Remove the basin and dry the arm, shoulder, and hand.
- Wash arm and hand closer to you in a similar manner.
- Place towel across chest and wash and rinse chest and breasts while lifting towel. Dry skin thoroughly and keep chest covered with towel.
- Wash, rinse, and dry abdomen.
- Change bathwater in basin, if needed, and get a clean washcloth.
- Expose the farther leg; flex leg and place bath towel lengthwise under the leg up to the buttocks.
- Wash, rinse, and dry leg and foot, making sure to dry between toes.
- Wash closer leg and foot in a similar manner.
- Perform toenail care.
- Assist client to turn on his or her side with back toward you.
- Fold a towel to expose back and buttocks, and place clean towel parallel to client's back.
- Wash, rinse, and dry the client's back and buttocks.
- Provide back rub using warmed lotion.
- Provide perineal care with clean washcloth and water.
- Place dirty linen in appropriate container.
- Remove gloves and wash hands.
- Make the client comfortable.
- Report and document anything unusual to the nurse.

Nursing Assistant/Nurse Aide Flash Review

PERINEAL CARE: FEMALES

PART
5

Perineal care is given during daily care and after the client defecates or urinates.

- Gather equipment.
- Wash hands and put on gloves.
- Provide privacy with a curtain, screen, or door.
- Check water temperature for safety and comfort.
- Place pad or linen protector under perineal area.
- Expose perineal area without overexposing client.
- Apply soap to wet washcloth and wash genital area from front to back using a clean part of the washcloth with each stroke.
- Rinse soap from genital area from front to back with a clean washcloth.
- Dry genital area from front to back with towel.
- Turn client on side and wash and rinse anal area from front to back.
- Dry anal area from front to back with towel.
- Reposition client.
- Dispose of soiled linen and clean basin.
- Remove gloves and wash hands.

PERINEAL CARE: MALES

. . . .

Perineal care is given during daily care and after the client defecates or urinates.

- Gather equipment.

- Wash hands and put on gloves.

- Provide privacy.

- Assist client to lie on back or side with a towel or bedpan under his hips.

- Fill basin with warm water, and cover client with a towel or sheet.

- Expose perineal area, and using a circular motion, gently wash the penis, cleaning from the tip downward. If the client is not circumcised, gently pull back the foreskin and wash the head of the penis. When finished, gently push the foreskin back into place. Rinse and dry the area.

- Wash and rinse the scrotum and the skin between the legs.

- Wash and rinse the anal area.

- Gently dry the perineal area.

- Remove towel or sheet.

- Remove gloves and wash hands.

- Report and record unusual findings to the nurse.

. . . .

Nursing Assistant/Nurse Aide Flash Review

FOOT CARE

. . . .

NAIL CARE

. . . .

- Wash hands and put on gloves.
- Explain procedure to client.
- Sit client in chair if possible. If client is on bed rest, perform foot care by flexing the client's legs.
- Fill a washbasin with warm water.
- Put towel under the basin.
- Place client's feet in the basin to soak for about 15 to 20 minutes.
- Apply soap to washcloth and wash feet, including between toes.
- Dry feet thoroughly.
- Apply lotion to feet, avoiding spaces between toes.
- Report and document any unusual findings to the nurse.

· ·

Nails should be short, clean, and smooth, because dirty nails spread infection, and jagged nails can cause injury. Lack of foot care for the elderly and those with poor circulation or diabetes can result in infection and even loss of a foot. To perform nail care, the nursing assistant should:

- Fill a washbasin with warm water and place a towel under the basin.
- Place the client's hands or feet in the basin to soak them for about 10 minutes.
- Gently push the cuticles back with a nail care stick while soaking the other hand or foot.
- Clean under the nails with a nail care stick.
- Trim the nails with a clipper, and file the edges with a nail file so that they are smooth—but do so only after getting permission and instructions from the nurse.
- Repeat the procedure for the other hand or foot.
- Dry the hands or feet fully, including between the fingers or toes.
- Apply lotion to the hands and feet but avoid the areas between the toes.

When doing foot care, with or without cutting the toenails, observe, clean, and dry all parts of the foot, including between the toes. Report and document the following: blue or pale nail beds, broken nails, bleeding, corns, or bunions.

· ·

SHAVING A CLIENT

. . . .

Shaving (male beard, female legs) is typically a client's choice. However, check with the nurse to make sure shaving is safe, because some clients have bleeding disorders and others are on medications that can cause bleeding problems.

- Gather all the needed supplies, and do not share shaving supplies between clients.

- Wash hands and put on gloves.

- Put a towel or other protective barrier under the area to be shaved.

- Follow the instructions for an electric razor; put warm water on the beard or hair to make it soft if using a regular razor.

- If needed, shake the shaving cream can, squirt some shaving cream on the nursing assistant's hand, and use it to lather the client's hair or beard.

- Hold the skin tight so that it is firm, and carefully shave a small area at a time, going in the same direction as the hair grows. When using a regular razor, rinse it after shaving each section.

- Rinse the razor and repeat the preceding step until the entire area is done.

- Wash and dry the shaved area, and apply lotion or aftershave if the client requests it.

- Remove gloves and wash hands.

If any bleeding occurs, apply pressure to the area, and report and document it.

. . . .

Nursing Assistant/Nurse Aide Flash Review

BACK RUBS

. . . .

Back rubs stimulate circulation, relax muscles, and refresh the client. When providing a back rub, the nursing assistant should:

• Warm the skin lotion in warm water.

• Wash hands using warm water.

• Apply gloves if the client has a rash or open cuts or sores on the back.

• Place the client on his or her side or abdomen.

• Put the lotion on the palms of both hands and rub to further warm lotion.

• Apply the lotion to the client's back with the palms of the hands, starting at the base of the spine and, using long, smooth strokes, move up to and around the shoulders and then down the sides of the back.

This should not be a deep muscle massage, and the nursing assistant should avoid using the fingertips or pinching muscles.

• •

HANDLING LINENS

. . . .

Bed making linens vary per facility. However, linens should be collected in the order in which they will be used. Linens can act as fomites, objects that can transmit infection. When handling linens, nursing assistants should:

- Always wash hands before collecting linens.

- Avoid holding clean or dirty linens next to their clothing.

- Collect only what is needed for a specific client's bed.

- Place clean linens on a clean surface.

- Wear gloves when removing linens from a bed.

- Roll linens toward the center of the bed when removing them.

- Clean mattress with an appropriate cleaning solution if bodily fluids have leaked onto mattress.

- Place dirty linens in the hamper immediately.

UNOCCUPIED (CLOSED) BED

. . . .

PART
5

Clean, wrinkle-free linens help prevent pressure ulcers and infections. To make an unoccupied (closed) bed, the nursing assistant should:

- Obtain supplies.

- Arrange the linens on a chair in the order in which they will be used.

- Adjust bed to appropriate height and lock wheels.

- Remove soiled linens by rolling them into a compact bundle, and place in hamper.

- Perform hand hygiene.

- Unfold bottom sheet on bed and tuck it under mattress to fit tightly and smoothly at head of the bed. Use mitered corners.

- Place draw sheet at center of bed and tuck it under mattress tightly and smoothly.

- Unfold top sheet on mattress wrong side up with hem even with top edge of mattress.

- Place the spread or blanket on the bed right side up with the top edge even with the top edge of the mattress, allowing it to hang evenly over the sides of the bed.

- Tuck top sheet and blanket as one unit under foot of mattress, using mitered corners.

- Fold the top sheet over the blanket to make an even cuff.

- Place case on pillow.

- Lower the bed back to its lowest position.

- Perform hand hygiene.

Nursing Assistant/Nurse Aide Flash Review

OCCUPIED BED

. . . .

When clients cannot get out of bed, the nursing assistant will make the bed with the client in it. This is usually done after the client is bathed and when linens become soiled. To make an occupied bed, the nursing assistant should:

- Explain procedure.

- Promote privacy.

- Lower head of bed before moving client.

- Make sure that client is covered with bath blanket while linens are changed.

- Loosen top linen from the end of the bed.

- Raise side rail on side where client will move.

- Assist client in moving/rolling toward rail.

- Loosen bottom used linen on working side and move bottom used linen toward center of bed.

- Place and tuck in clean bottom linen on working side and tuck it under client.

- Assist client with moving/rolling onto clean bottom linen.

- Raise side rail and go to other side of bed.

- Remove used bottom linen.

- Tighten and tuck in clean bottom linen, making sure it is free of wrinkles.

- Cover client with clean top sheet and remove bath blanket.

- Change pillowcase.

- Dispose of used linens into hamper; do not place on floor.

- Make sure call bell is within the client's reach.

- Wash hands.

. . . .

ADMISSIONS

. . . .

TRANSFERS

. . . .

PART
5

The admission is the client's official entry into the hospital or other facility. Admission is frequently stressful for both the client and the family. The nursing assistant is usually responsible for helping client unpack; taking and documenting vital signs, height, and weight; helping client change into the hospital gown; and making sure the client is comfortable. To help the client feel welcome, the nursing assistant should:

• Prepare the room before the client arrives.

• Greet the client and introduce self.

• Use good communication skills.

• Help the person settle into the new room, demonstrating the use of the call bell, bed, lights, and other appliances and equipment.

• Complete a resident inventory record if the client is admitted to long-term care.

. . . .

Clients are sometimes moved within or between healthcare facilities. The nursing assistant's duties for transfers will vary by facility. In some cases, the nursing assistant will be responsible for packing the client's belongings and ensuring that they are transferred with the client so that nothing is lost. The nursing assistant may also assist with the physical transfer of the client. In long-term care facilities, nursing assistants will also be responsible for reporting client personal care information to the receiving nursing assistant.

. . . .

DISCHARGES

. . . .

PART
5

The discharge is the official release of a client from the facility after the client's discharge is ordered by the physician. Some clients may choose to leave against medical advice (AMA), which is permissible for mentally competent clients. Discharge planning actually begins when the client is admitted, with the goal of the client having the best possible health outcome after leaving the facility. Discharge teaching (instructions for postdischarge personal care) can be considerable, and the client may have difficulty with it. The nursing assistant should report any of the following to the nurse:

- changes in the client's mental status or vital signs
- questions about the client's condition
- comments that suggest the client or family members do not understand discharge teaching
- signs of anxiety
- any mention that a client wishes to sign out AMA

Nursing Assistant/Nurse Aide Flash Review

DRESSING CLIENT WITH A WEAK OR AFFECTED ARM

. . . .

- Wash hands.

- Provide privacy.

- Ask client which top he or she would like to wear, and respect the choice unless contraindicated.

- Remove gown from the unaffected side first, then from the affected side, making sure to avoid overexposing client.

- Assist client in placing the affected or weak arm through the appropriate sleeve of the top before placing garment on the unaffected arm.

- Throughout the procedure, carefully move the client to avoid overextending the client's limbs and joints.

- Finish with clothing in place and make sure call bell is within the client's reach.

- Place soiled gown into soiled linen container.

- Wash hands.

. . . .

HAIR CARE

Routine hair care is part of daily personal care, and clients should be encouraged to participate in their own care as much as possible. When caring for a client's hair and scalp, the nursing assistant should report any redness, flaking, or crusting of the scalp; itching or tenderness; unusual hair loss; foul odor; severely matted hair; or lice eggs (nits). When shampooing a client's hair in bed, the nursing assistant will:

- Cover the pillow with a towel or protective cover to keep it dry.

- Untie the client's gown and place a towel under the person's neck and arms.

- Place the shampoo pan under the person's head.

- Place a washcloth over the person's eyes so the shampoo does not hurt them.

- Use warm water and pour a small amount on the hair using a water pitcher; keep as much water as possible off the face.

- Put a small amount of shampoo on the head and gently massage the hair and scalp with fingertips.

- Rinse the head with water, starting at the top of the head and letting the water work its way down to the bottom.

- Repeat shampoo and rinse as needed.

- Help the client into a sitting position if permissible.

- Dry hair with blow-dryer if possible.

- Change the client's gown if needed.

- Assist client into a comfortable position.

HAND CARE

. . . .

APPLYING MAKEUP

. . . .

PROSTHETIC AND ORTHOTIC DEVICES

PART 5

Some clients require assistance caring for their own hands. To do this, the nursing assistant will:

- Check water temperature.
- Place basin on towel or protective pad at comfortable height for client, providing support for forearm if elbow is raised during the procedure.
- Place hand in water for five minutes.
- Wash top and bottom of hand and between fingers.
- Use fresh cloth to rinse.
- Dry hand, including between fingers, and rest hand on towel.
- Remove residue under nails with nail care stick, cleaning edge of stick on towel between each nail.
- Complete procedure with the other hand.
- Apply lotion from fingertips to wrists.
- Clean equipment.
- Wash hands.

· ·

Helping clients maintain their normal grooming can increase their sense of well-being. When helping a client with makeup application, realize that some clients may use styles that were popular in their younger years.

· ·

Some clients use special prosthetic or other devices, including artificial limbs. Report any skin abnormalities, such as redness, pain, or ulceration, to the nurse.

· ·

BASIC POSITIONS

Clients are placed in different positions, usually to allow access to different parts of the body. Regardless of position, the nursing assistant should ensure that the client's dignity and privacy are maintained. Curtains and doors should be closed, and the client should be adequately draped with a sheet or blanket.

Position	Description	Examples of Use
Prone	Client is lying on stomach with knees straight.	Exams of posterior parts of the body
Supine	Client is lying on back with knees straight, and arms are at the sides.	Exams of anterior parts of the body
Side-lying	Client is positioned on right or left side.	To remove pressure off the back
Knee-chest	The client's head and chest are flat against the examining table, while the knees are bent; the client's weight is mainly on the knees and chest.	Rectal exam
Sims'	Client is lying partly on side and partly on back.	Administering rectal suppositories and enemas
Trendelenberg	Client is supine, and bed is tilted so that the client's head is below the level of the feet.	Shock
Fowler's	Client is sitting up in bed at a 45° to 90° angle.	Eating, reading
Semi-Fowler's	Client is sitting slightly at a 30° angle. It is mainly used to help promote a client's lung expansion.	Difficulty breathing; to prevent client from sliding down in bed
Lithotomy	Client is lying on back with knees bent, thighs apart, and feet resting in stirrups.	Pelvic exams
Dorsal recumbent	Client is lying on back with knees bent and feet flat on the examination table.	Abdominal exams

• •

Nursing Assistant/Nurse Aide Flash Review

COMPLICATIONS OF BED REST

....

Bed rest can be necessary for healing; however, extensive periods of bed rest can cause harm to the rest of the body. Complications of bed rest include:

- pressure ulcers
- muscle contractures
- loss of muscle strength
- bone loss
- kidney stones
- constipation
- decreased pulmonary functioning
- postural hypotension
- behavioral and emotional changes

The following symptoms of immobility complications should be reported to the nurse immediately:

- reddened areas on skin
- pale or shiny skin over a bone area
- breaks in the skin
- painful, red, and hot areas in the lower legs (do not rub these areas, as they may be signs of a blood clot and rubbing can cause an embolus)
- new urinary or bowel incontinence or retention
- new complaints of pain

APPLYING KNEE-HIGH ELASTIC STOCKING

. . . .

Antiembolism stockings are specially fitted stockings that compress the veins to help blood return to the heart and keep it from pooling in the legs. They may be ordered before or after surgery. To apply elastic stockings:

- Explain procedure.
- Wash hands.
- Assure privacy.
- Assist client into supine position.
- Turn stocking inside out.
- Place foot of stocking over toes, foot, and heel.
- Pull top of stocking over foot, heel, and leg.
- Carefully move foot and leg gently and naturally to avoid force and overextension of limb and joints.
- Make sure there are no twists or wrinkles and that the heel of stocking (if present) is over the heel and the opening in the toe area (if present) is either over or under the toe area.
- Wash hands.

GUIDELINES FOR POSITIONING CLIENTS

. . . .

Most clients require repositioning at least every two hours. Nursing assistants should be alert for complications of immobility whenever repositioning a client and should follow these guidelines:

- Plan ahead.
- Know the positioning care plan for clients under care.
- Always use good body mechanics.
- Get help when needed.
- Reposition every two hours or as ordered.
- Allow client to assist whenever possible.
- Provide for the client's dignity and privacy.
- Protect client's tubing from kinking or being pulled out.
- Be gentle.
- Do not move client by pulling on limbs.
- Check client's skin after repositioning.
- Make sure the bedding is wrinkle free after positioning.

. . . .

Nursing Assistant/Nurse Aide Flash Review

POSITIONING CLIENT ON SIDE

· ·

Clients may need positioning from side to side for personal comfort or to prevent postoperative complications such as pneumonia and embolism. To position the client on his or her side, the nursing assistant will:

- Explain procedure.

- Provide privacy.

- Wash hands.

- Raise bed to a comfortable level to provide care and lock it.

- Lower head of bed and raise side rail on side to which client will be turned.

- Slowly roll client onto side as one unit toward raised side rail.

- Place or adjust pillow under head for support.

- Position client properly so that he or she is not lying on arm.

- Support client's top arm with supportive device or pillow.

- Place supportive device or pillow behind client's back.

- Place supportive device or pillow between client's legs with top knee flexed, supporting knee and ankle.

- Lower bed and make sure call bell is within reach.

- Wash hands.

GUIDELINES FOR ASSISTING CLIENTS WITH TRANSFERS

. . . .

TRANSFER BELTS

. . . .

PART 5

The term *transfer* means moving a client from one place to another. When transferring clients, follow these general guidelines:

- Plan ahead.

- Know the transferring care plan for clients under care.

- Always use good body mechanics.

- Get help when needed.

- Have client lead with stronger side.

- Have client hold the chair or nursing assistant's arm for support; never let client hang on to nursing assistant's neck.

- Do not hold client under the arms.

- Check clothing and shoes for proper fit.

- Make sure bed, stretcher, or wheelchair is locked.

- Make sure bed is in its lowest position.

. . . .

A transfer belt is used to assist weak or unsteady clients with transferring, standing, and walking. It is sometimes referred to as a gait belt when used for ambulation. Transfer belts can be dangerous for certain clients, such as those who recently had abdominal surgery or those with certain heart disease. Therefore, the nursing assistant should check the care plan or check with the nurse before using one on a client.

. . . .

ASSISTING CLIENT TO AMBULATE USING TRANSFER BELT

. . . .

To use a transfer belt to ambulate a client, the nursing assistant should:

- Explain procedure.

- Wash hands.

- Before assisting client to stand:
    - Make sure client is wearing shoes.
    - Make sure bed is at a safe level.
    - Lock bed wheels.
    - Assist client into a sitting position with client's feet flat on the floor.
    - Apply transfer belt securely over client's clothing/gown.
    - Provide instructions to help client stand, including a prearranged signal to alert client to begin standing.

- Stand facing client and position self to ensure safety of client and self during transfer.

- Using prearranged signal, alert client to begin standing.

- Gradually assist client to stand by grasping transfer belt on both sides with an upward grasp, maintaining stability of client's legs.

- Walk slightly behind and to one side of client while holding on to the belt.

- After ambulation, assist client to bed and remove transfer belt.

- Wash hands.

. . . .

TRANSFERRING CLIENT FROM BED TO WHEELCHAIR USING TRANSFER BELT

PART 5

Wheelchairs can pose safety risks, and thus must be checked before use. To transfer a client from bed to wheelchair using transfer belt, the nursing assistant will:

- Explain procedure.

- Provide privacy.

- Before assisting the client to stand:
    - Position wheelchair at the side of bed, near the head of bed and facing the foot of the bed.
    - Make sure that footrests are folded up or removed.
    - Make sure that bed is at a safe level.
    - Lock wheels on wheelchair.
    - Assist client into a sitting position with feet flat on the floor.
    - Make sure client is wearing shoes.
    - Apply transfer belt securely over the client's clothing/gown.
    - Provide instructions to help client transfer, including a prearranged signal to alert client to begin transfer.

- Stand facing client and position self to ensure safety of client and self during transfer.

- Using prearranged signal, alert client to begin standing.

- Gradually assist client to stand by grasping transfer belt on both sides with an upward grasp, maintaining stability of client's legs.

- Assist client in turning to stand in front of wheelchair, making sure that back of client's legs are against the wheelchair.

- Lower client into chair and position so that hips touch back of wheelchair.

- Remove transfer belt.

- Position feet on footrests.

- Make sure that client is adequately covered to preserve client's modesty.

- Provide call bell.

Nursing Assistant/Nurse Aide Flash Review

CONTRACTURES

. . . .

RANGE OF MOTION EXERCISES

. . . .

A contracture is abnormal shortening of muscle due to immobility. It makes the muscle highly resistant to passive stretching.

. . . .

Range of motion (ROM) exercises put joints through their complete pain-free range of motion to preserve joint and muscle functioning in clients who have limited musculoskeletal functioning. Types are:

- Active-assisted range of motion exercises are generally performed by the client with some assistance from a physical therapist or other health-care provider.

- Active range of motion exercises can be performed by client under the guidance and direction of a physical therapist or other healthcare provider.

- Passive range of motion exercises are done completely by the physical therapist or healthcare provider for clients who are paralyzed or too weak to perform movement on their own.

Nursing assistants help clients with passive range of motion exercises during their bath or dressing routine. Bed-bound clients should have range of motion exercises at least once a day to prevent contractures.

. . . .

PASSIVE RANGE OF MOTION FOR KNEE AND ANKLE

. . . .

PASSIVE RANGE OF MOTION FOR SHOULDERS

. . . .

To perform passive range of motion for knee and ankle:

- Wash hands.

- Explain procedure.

- Provide privacy.

- Tell client to let nursing assistant know if pain occurs during the exercise.

- Support leg at knee and ankle while performing exercise.

- Flex and extend knee at least three times unless client complains of pain.

- Support foot and ankle close to bed.

- Dorsiflex (pull foot up toward head) and plantar flex (pull foot down toward floor) at least three times.

- Always move joints slowly and gently, and stop if client complains of pain.

- Wash hands.

. . . .

To perform passive range of motion for shoulders:

- Wash hands.

- Explain procedure.

- Provide privacy.

- Tell client to let nursing assistant know if pain occurs during the exercise.

- Support client's arm at elbow and wrist while performing range of motion for shoulder.

- Raise client's straightened arm upward toward head to ear level and return arm down to side of body at least three times unless client complains of pain.

- Repeat with other arm and shoulder.

- Always move joints slowly and gently, and stop if client complains of pain.

- Wash hands.

. . . .

DANGLING (SITTING ON THE EDGE OF THE BED)

A person who has been lying down for a long while may become dizzy and unsteady when attempting to stand. Dangling (sitting at the edge of the bed) for a while allows a person to gain one's balance before standing. To assist a person with dangling:

- Wash hands.

- Explain procedure.

- Provide privacy.

- Place bed in low position and lock the bed wheels.

- Raise side rail on side opposite of where client will sit.

- Place the client in supine position and raise the head of the bed to about 45°.

- Assist client in swinging his or her legs to the side while raising shoulders off the bed.

- Assist client into a sitting position and support client's shoulders.

- Allow client to gain balance while sitting on the side of the bed, and be prepared to assist client back into a supine position if the client becomes dizzy or feels faint.

- When client feels sturdy enough to sit unassisted, remove your hands from his or her shoulder and allow client to sit at the side of the bed.

- Then either assist client to a standing position or back to a supine position.

- Ensure that client is comfortable and that the call bell is within reach.

- Wash hands.

- Report to the nurse how long client tolerated sitting, how well the client tolerated sitting, and if there were any problems.

. . . .

Nursing Assistant/Nurse Aide Flash Review

HYDRATION AND FLUID BALANCE

. . . .

DEHYDRATION

. . . .

FLUID INTAKE

PART
5

Water is critical for life. Approximately half of an adult's total body weight is fluid, while 70% to 80% of an infant's body weight is water. Fluid balance is the balance of the input and output of fluids in the body. Fluid balance is important for homeostasis, which is the body's way of keeping itself in a stable state. Fluid imbalance occurs when the body retains or loses too much fluid or when the body does not get adequate fluid.

• •

Dehydration occurs when the body does not have adequate fluid; it can be caused by a number of problems, including vomiting, diarrhea, bleeding, and wound drainage.

• •

The average adult takes in three quarts (3,312 ml) of fluid each day by drinking liquids, and to some extent, consuming food. Clients may also receive fluids via intravenous (parenteral intake) tubes or nasogastric (enteral intake) tubes.

FLUID OUTPUT

. . . .

INTAKE AND OUTPUT (I&O)

. . . .

MEASURING ORAL FLUID INTAKE

PART
5

Fluid output is the total of fluids that exit the body via urination (voiding), perspiration (sweating), evaporation (breathing), and stooling. Fluid output should equal fluid intake, and thus people eliminate three quarts (3,312 ml) of fluid each day.

. . . .

Tell clients that you are measuring their intake and output (I&O) so that they can assist in the process. However, it is the nursing assistant's responsibility to assess the oral fluid intake and the output.

. . . .

Oral fluids include all liquids (water, soda, juice, milk, etc.) and semisolids such as gelatin and ice cream. Oral fluid intake is usually measured in cubic centimeters (cc), and it is critical that nursing assistants observe the exact amounts of fluids taken in by clients and that they record the amounts accurately.

MEASURING AND RECORDING URINARY OUTPUT

. . . .

NPO

. . . .

RESTRICTED FLUIDS

- Put on clean gloves.

- Pour contents of bedpan into measuring container without spilling or splashing urine.

- Measure the amount of urine by examining it at eye level with container on flat surface.

- Note amount.

- Empty contents of measuring container into toilet.

- Rinse measuring container and pour rinse water into toilet.

- Rinse bedpan and pour rinse water into toilet.

- Remove and dispose of gloves without contaminating self.

- Wash hands.

- Record output on intake and output record within plus or minus 25 ml/cc of nurse's reading.

. . . .

NPO (*nil per os*) means nothing by mouth, and thus the client in NPO status is not allowed to have anything to drink or eat. Some may not even be allowed to have oral hygiene. They should not have a water pitcher by their bedside and should have an NPO sign over their bed. Physicians order NPO status and usually do so before certain tests and surgery. NPO status can create stress for the client, and thus, the nursing assistant should provide reassurance.

. . . .

Clients may be placed on fluid restriction due to certain illnesses. When caring for a client on fluid restriction, the nursing assistant should place a Restricted Fluids sign above the client's bed, remind client about the fluid restriction, and accurately record the client's fluid intake.

NUTRIENTS

. . . .

NUTRITIONAL ASSESSMENT

. . . .

CULTURAL AND RELIGIOUS CONSIDERATIONS

PART
5

A well-balanced diet consists of fruits, grains, vegetables, and protein. The six essential nutrients are:

1. Carbohydrates are starch, fiber, and various sugars. Healthy sources of carbohydrates include grain breads, muesli, cereals, potatoes, brown pasta, brown rice, fruits, and vegetables.

2. Fats are saturated, unsaturated, and polyunsaturated fatty acids. They are needed for energy and for the body to be able to absorb fat-soluble vitamins (vitamins A, D, E, and K). Good fats include oily fish, yogurt, and cheese.

3. Proteins are needed for all cells, tissues, and hormone productions. The chief sources of protein are meat, fish, eggs, legumes, and dairy products.

4. Water is needed for all body functions and comes from liquids and foods.

5. Vitamins are needed for normal metabolism, growth, development, and regulation of cell function. There are fat-soluble vitamins (vitamins A, D, E, and K) and water-soluble vitamins (multiple vitamin B and vitamin C).

6. Minerals are formed by plants or animals and are needed for healthy bones, teeth, and blood, as well as normal heart rhythm, cellular metabolism, and muscle reflexes.

· ·

Nursing assistants observe for and report any problems with a client's nutritional status. These may include inadequate food intake, chewing or swallowing difficulties, nausea, vomiting, diarrhea, constipation, and weight changes.

· ·

Many clients have specific food restrictions and/or preferences because of their religion or culture. Therefore, the nursing assistant should be aware of these and respect them. Family members may bring in food items and should be allowed to do so, unless the items are not allowed due to the client's medical condition.

Nursing Assistant/Nurse Aide Flash Review

DIETARY ISSUES FOR SENIORS

. . . .

SPECIAL DIETS

. . . .

ASSISTING A CLIENT WITH EATING

PART 5

Dietary issues for seniors include loss of appetite, reduced sense of taste, tooth loss, denture problems, dehydration, malnutrition, and severe weight loss or gain.

. . . .

Special diets include:

- regular: well-balanced variety of foods
- bland: mild foods, no spices, alcohol, or caffeine
- low-calorie: low calories for weight loss
- diabetic: individualized diet with accurate balance of carbohydrates, proteins, and fats
- soft: foods soft in consistency and no strong flavors
- mechanical soft: same as soft but food is ground and pureed
- low-residue: no fiber, bulk, or seeds
- high-residue: high fiber
- low-sodium: no salt on tray; limited foods that contain sodium
- gluten-free: no foods that contain gluten
- full fluids: all mild liquids plus semisolids like ice cream and soup
- clear liquids: clear fluids, no milk

. . . .

Clients usually look forward to mealtime, and selecting their own food choices gives them a greater sense of independence. The nursing assistant should do whatever is possible to make mealtime pleasant.

Nursing Assistant/Nurse Aide Flash Review

FEEDING CLIENT WHO CANNOT FEED SELF

....

USING ASSISTIVE DEVICES FOR FEEDING

....

INTRAVENOUS (IV) THERAPY

PART 5

- Wash hands.
- Ensure that client is receiving the correct meal/food items by checking the name on the tray or items.
- Assist client into upright sitting position (45° to 90°).
- Assist client with cleaning hands before eating.
- Place tray where client can see it.
- Sit facing client.
- Explain what foods are on tray and ask which one the client would like to eat first.
- Use a spoon and offer the client one bite of each type of food on tray, describing the content of each spoonful.
- Offer beverage during meal.
- Ensure that client's mouth is empty before offering next bite of food or sip of beverage.
- When finished, wipe client's mouth and hands.
- Remove food tray and place tray in designated area.
- Wash hands.
- Report and record client's intake as needed.

. . . .

Some clients may need assistive devices for eating and drinking. If a client uses such devices, the nursing assistant should learn how to use the device as needed.

. . . .

Intravenous (IV) therapy is the administration of fluids, medications, and/or nutrients into a vein. When caring for a client who is receiving IV, check the solution, tubing, and drip chamber. Also note the skin at the catheter site and report any redness, swelling, or bleeding.

ENTERAL NUTRITION

. . . .

TOTAL PARENTERAL NUTRITION (TPN)

. . . .

PART
5

Enteral feedings are provided through a nasogastric tube or a gastrostomy tube.

• Nasogastric tubes are inserted by the nurse or the physician through the client's nose down into the stomach. The tubes are used for gastric suctioning or short-term tube feeding. The nursing assistant's responsibility for nasogastric tubes varies by state.

• Gastrostomy tubes are inserted through an opening into the stomach via the abdomen while the client is under anesthesia. They are used for clients who are unable to eat through the mouth.

Tube feedings may be intermittent or continuous. The tube feedings should be warmed to room temperature, and the tube should be checked for correct placement before the feeding is started.

· ·

Total parenteral nutrition (TPN) is the infusion of fluids and nutrients via a catheter placed in a central or peripheral vein. This is used when clients cannot receive enteral feedings and is associated with several possible complications, including infection.

· ·

NORMAL URINATION

. . . .

URINE COLOR AND CHARACTERISTICS

. . . .

URINARY INCONTINENCE

PART 5

Urine acts as part of the body's disposal process by removing the extra water and water-soluble wastes the kidneys filter from the blood.

. . . .

COLOR AND CHARACTERISTICS	URINE
Clear straw yellow	Normal urine
Cloudy	Infection
Dark brown	Liver disorder
Pink, red, light brown	Beets, food coloring, blood disorder, bleeding in the urinary tract
Dark yellow or orange	B vitamins, certain medications, laxative use
Blue or green	Artificial colorings, medications, infection

. . . .

Urinary incontinence is the loss of bladder control. The severity ranges from occasionally leaking urine when coughing and sneezing to frequent wetting. Incontinence may be due to muscle or nerve damage (stress or overflow incontinence), mental conditions such as Alzheimer's disease or stroke, and inability to get to the toilet in time (functional incontinence). When caring for a client with urinary incontinence, the nursing assistant should check the client frequently for wetness, clean and change the client as needed, and observe for signs of skin breakdown. This condition can also be embarrassing, so the nursing assistant should also provide support.

URINARY RETENTION

. . . .

URINARY CATHETERS

. . . .

PROVIDING CATHETER CARE FOR FEMALES

Urinary retention is the inability to urinate. It can be acute or chronic and can range from incomplete bladder emptying to total lack of voiding. Some clients with this condition may have overflow incontinence.

· ·

A urinary catheter is a tube that is inserted into the urethra and bladder to drain urine from the body. Catheters may be used for one urine withdrawal or left in place for days or weeks. Long-term catheters are used for urinary retention and to keep incontinent clients dry.

· ·

When providing urinary catheter care for female clients:

- Explain procedure.

- Provide privacy.

- Wash hands and put on gloves.

- Check water temperature for safety and comfort.

- Place linen protector under perineal area before washing.

- Expose area surrounding catheter but avoid overexposure of client.

- Apply soap to wet washcloth.

- Hold catheter near meatus without tugging, and clean at least four inches of catheter nearest meatus, moving only away from meatus and using a clean area of the cloth for each stroke.

- Hold catheter near meatus without tugging and dry four inches of catheter, moving away from meatus.

- Empty, rinse, and dry basin, and place it in dirty supply area.

- Dispose of used linen into soiled linen container.

- Remove gloves.

- Wash hands.

Nursing Assistant/Nurse Aide Flash Review

EMPTYING THE CATHETER BAG

· ·

Urine is removed from the bag to measure it and clear the bag.

- Gather equipment.
- Wash hands and put on gloves.
- Unbend kinks in catheter tubing.
- Make sure catheter bag is hanging lower than the bladder.
- Open drain on bottom of bag and let urine run into graduated container.
- Once bag is empty, close drain, wipe it with an alcohol wipe, and return it to the holder.
- Measure the urine amount.
- Record the amount on the intake and output record.

. . . .

ASSISTING CLIENTS WITH BEDPANS

· ·

PART 5

- Wash hands and put on gloves.
- Provide privacy.
- Raise bed rails on the opposite side of the bed.
- Raise bed to a comfortable working position.
- Apply powder to the bedpan.
- Fold back sheets and lift the client's gown.
- Have client bend knees and raise hips, put a protective pad on the bed, and place the bedpan against the client's buttocks. If the client is unable to raise hips, turn the client on his or her side, place the bedpan against the buttocks, and turn client onto back with the bedpan under the buttocks.
- Cover the client.
- Raise head of bed to sitting position.
- Place call bell and toilet tissue within reach and instruct client to call when finished.
- Raise side rail.
- Dispose of gloves and wash hands.
- Return when client signals.
- Wash hands and put on gloves.
- Help client raise hips and remove bedpan, or lower the head of the bed, hold the bedpan, and remove it as client rolls off it.
- Cover pan.
- Assist client if she cannot clean self.
- Remove protective pad and lower the bed.
- Clean bedpan by following the facility's policy.
- Discard gloves and wash hands.

. . . .

Nursing Assistant/Nurse Aide Flash Review

ASSISTING CLIENTS WITH URINALS

. . . .

- Wash hands and put on gloves.
- Provide privacy.
- Give client the urinal and ask him to signal when finished.
- Dispose of gloves and wash hands.
- When client signals, wash hands and put on gloves.
- Take urinal, cover it, and bring it to bathroom.
- Check urine and measure it.
- Clean urinal according to facility policy.
- Remove gloves and wash hands.

. . . .

NORMAL BOWEL ELIMINATION

. . . .

STOOL COLOR AND CHARACTERISTICS

. . . .

BOWEL INCONTINENCE

PART 5

The frequency, amount, and characteristics of bowel movements differ from person to person, as bowel movements are affected by several factors, including fluid intake, diet, medications, and activity level. Nursing assistants should know their clients' bowel patterns so that they will also be aware of any changes to these patterns.

. . . .

COLOR	POSSIBLE CAUSE
Green	Diarrhea, green food coloring, green vegetables
Pale or clay colored	Bile duct obstruction, certain medications
Yellow, greasy, and foul	Fat in stool, malabsorption
Black	Bleeding in upper gastrointestinal (GI) tract, iron supplements
Bright red	Bleeding in lower GI tract; iron supplements

. . . .

Bowel incontinence is the inability to hold feces. It can be temporary or permanent, and can be caused by diarrhea or inability to get to the bathroom in time. Unconscious persons will also be incontinent. Bowel training may assist some clients, and all clients should be kept clean and dry and observed for skin breakdown.

ENEMAS

. . . .

RECTAL SUPPOSITORIES

. . . .

OSTOMY CARE

PART 5

Enemas are used to flush fluid into the colon to remove stool from the rectum. They are used to treat constipation and fecal impactions and to cleanse the colon before surgery or procedures. They include:

- cleansing enemas that contain water, soapsuds, or saline

- oil retention enemas that contain mineral, olive, or cottonseed oil

- commercial enemas that contain solutions to irritate the bowel to cause peristalsis and soften the stool

Enemas are usually given by a nurse, but some facilities allow nursing assistants to administer them. They are given with the client on the left side in Sims' position.

• •

Rectal suppositories are waxlike bullet-shaped substances that contain medications, usually for constipation or fever. These are administered by the nurse.

• •

An ostomy is a surgically created way for people to eliminate stool, usually because the person had a tumor or significant intestinal problem. The nursing assistant's role in ostomy care is determined by the facility; however, all nursing assistants should observe the skin around the ostomy for signs of breakdown.

PAIN RESPONSE

. . . .

NONVERBAL SIGNS OF PAIN

. . . .

PAIN ASSESSMENT

Pain can range from discomfort to severe suffering. It can be acute or chronic and can be caused by several factors, including trauma, illness, and surgery.

- Pain threshold: The pain threshold is the point when the person becomes aware of pain.

- Pain tolerance: Pain tolerance is the level of pain a person can tolerate before seeking help.

. . . .

Nonverbal signs of pain include crying, facial expressions, moaning, restlessness, sweating, and guarding the painful area.

. . . .

When assessing pain, the nursing assistant should get the following information:

- Location of the pain: where it is and where it radiates to.

- Severity of the pain: a pain scale of 0 to 10 can be used.

- Characteristics of the pain: description of the pain (sharp, dull, stabbing, etc.).

- Circumstances: when pain started, whether the client had this pain before, what makes it worse, what makes it better.

TREATMENTS FOR PAIN

. . . .

NURSING ASSISTANT ROLE IN PAIN MANAGEMENT

. . . .

HEAT APPLICATION

PART 5

Pain can be treated with medications or alternative measures, including transcutaneous electric nerve stimulation (TENS), which delivers electric impulses to help block pain signals.

. . . .

To assist clients in pain, the nursing assistant can help the person relax, provide distractions, position for better comfort, massage the area if not prohibited, and be slow and gentle with care.

. . . .

Heat applications are used to reduce pain and swelling, relieve muscle spasms, and provide warmth. Dry heat prevents moisture from coming into contact with the skin and includes hot water bottles and heating pads. Moist heat works faster and deeper than dry heat, and thus, is used at lower temperatures.

Nursing Assistant/Nurse Aide Flash Review

DRY HEAT APPLICATION WITH AN AQUAMATIC PAD

. . . .

COLD APPLICATIONS

. . . .

PART
5

To use dry heat application with an aquamatic pad:

- Make sure pad and its electrical cord are in good working condition.

- Fill pad with distilled water if needed; do not use tap water.

- Keep heating unit level with tubing and pad.

- Allow the water to warm to the desired temperature per order, and place pad inside cover.

- Place bed at comfortable working height.

- Assist client into comfortable position.

- Expose only the area to be treated.

- Apply pad to site.

- Leave pad in place for the amount of time ordered.

- Check skin under pad every five minutes. Discontinue pad and report to nurse if skin becomes red, swollen, painful, numb, or blistered.

- Refill with water if needed.

- When treatment is complete, remove the pad, straighten the bed linens, and make sure client is comfortable and in good alignment.

- Set bed at lowest position.

- Wash hands.

. . . .

Cold applications are used to reduce pain, control bleeding, numb sensation, and relieve fever. They are also used for musculoskeletal trauma because they reduce pain and swelling. Moist cold applications penetrate more quickly and deeply; dry applications are usually colder. Cold applications can also cause blistering and thus, should be handled with care.

. . . .

Nursing Assistant/Nurse Aide Flash Review

MOIST COLD APPLICATION

. . . .

DRY COLD APPLICATION

. . . .

PART 5

To use moist cold applications:

- Put ice in the bath basin and fill the basin with cold water.
- Set bed at comfortable working height.
- Lock wheels.
- Use linen protector to keep bed dry.
- Moisten compress in ice water and wring it out.
- Apply compress for prescribed amount of time.
- Keep it moist with ice water and check skin every 10 minutes. Discontinue treatment if area becomes numb, pale, or blue, and report this to the nurse.
- Remove compress when treatment time is over.
- Remove linen protector and straighten linens.
- Lower bed to lowest position and lock wheels.
- Dispose of soiled linens and clean equipment.
- Wash hands.

. . . .

To apply dry cold application:

- Fill the ice bag with water and check for leaks. Empty the bag and fill it one-half to two-thirds full with crushed ice; do not overfill it. Squeeze out excess air, and dry bag.
- Position bed at comfortable working height and lock wheels.
- Assist person into comfortable position.
- Apply ice bag to site and leave on for prescribed time
- Check skin every 10 minutes. Discontinue treatment if area becomes numb, pale, or blue, and report this to the nurse.
- Refill bag with ice as needed.
- Remove bag at end of the prescribed time.
- Straighten linens and make sure client is comfortable.
- Lower bed to lowest position and lock wheels.
- Dispose of soiled linens and clean equipment.
- Wash hands.

. . . .

NORMAL SLEEP

. . . .

THE SLEEP CYCLE

. . . .

SLEEP REQUIREMENTS

PART 5

Sleep enables the body to rest and restore its energy. Healthy sleep helps people cope with stress, solve problems, or recover from illness. The blood pressure, temperature, pulse, and respirations are lower during sleep. People also need rest, which is a state where people feel comfortable, calm, and free of anxiety.

· ·

The sleep cycle consists of two basic states: rapid eye movement (REM) sleep and nonrapid eye movement (NREM) sleep. Sleep usually begins with non-REM sleep.

- REM sleep usually occurs about 90 minutes after falling asleep. The first period of REM sleep lasts about 10 minutes, and each recurring REM stage increases in time, with the final one lasting about an hour. Dreams usually occur in the REM stage.

- Non-REM sleep is made up of four stages, each lasting 5 to 15 minutes. These stages progress from light to very deep sleep.

· ·

The amount of sleep each person needs is individualized; however, on average, adults sleep seven to eight hours per day, older adults about five to six hours, teenagers about nine hours per day, and infants about 16 to 18 hours per day.

· ·

Nursing Assistant/Nurse Aide Flash Review

FACTORS THAT CAUSE SLEEP PROBLEMS

. . . .

SLEEP LOSS

. . . .

INSOMNIA

PART 5

Factors that cause sleep problems include illness, pain, stress, depression, anxiety, alcohol, caffeine, genetics, certain medications, noises in the environment, exercise two hours or less before sleeping, strange bed, and aging.

. . . .

Sleep loss can result in worsened pain, decreased immune response, increased risk for illness, slowed healing process, emotional and behavioral problems, decreased cognition, impaired memory, fatigue, and decreased work ability.

. . . .

Insomnia is a disorder in which people have difficulty falling asleep, staying asleep, or both. Sleep quality is poor; insomniacs wake up feeling tired, and this affects their ability to function during the day. Nursing assistants should tell the nurse if clients complain of insomnia so that it can be assessed and treated.

SLEEP APNEA

. . . .

NURSING ASSISTANT ROLE IN PROMOTING SLEEP AND REST

. . . .

PART 5

Sleep apnea is a disorder in which a person stops breathing for periods of time during sleep. There are different types of sleep apnea, but the most common is obstructive. In obstructive sleep apnea, the soft tissue in the back of the throat collapses, blocks the airway, and causes breathing to stop. When the person's oxygen level gets low, he or she wakes up and starts breathing again. These constant disruptions make sleep quality poor. The person feels tired and has trouble staying awake during the day.

Sleep apnea is most common in overweight men over age 40, and symptoms include loud chronic snoring, gasping and choking during sleep, excessive sleepiness in the day, and possibly mood and cognitive changes. Treatment includes weight loss, alcohol and smoking avoidance, and avoiding certain sleep positions. Surgery may be possible. Some clients are treated with continuous positive airway pressure (CPAP) therapy, in which the person wears a special mask while sleeping. The mask is connected to a machine that keeps the person's oxygen at an adequate level.

When caring for a client who uses CPAP, the nursing assistant may need to help the client with putting on the mask and cleaning the equipment.

· ·

To help promote sleep, the nursing assistant can:

• Encourage increased activity during the day.

• Limit naps.

• Avoid giving the client caffeinated beverages in the afternoon or evening.

• Offer a warm drink.

• Promote evening relaxation with a warm bath and massage.

• Create a comfortable environment, including low lighting.

• Play low, soft music.

• Position client for good body alignment.

• Avoid waking client up for vital signs if possible.

· ·

REPORTING SLEEP DIFFICULTIES

. . . .

Nursing assistants should record and report the following:

- Client frequently awakes during the night.
- Client has trouble falling asleep.
- Client reports problems sleeping.
- Client gets up frequently at night to urinate.

. . . .

PURPOSE OF COLLECTING SPECIMENS

. . . .

STANDARD PRECAUTIONS

. . . .

ASEPTIC TECHNIQUE

PART 5

Specimens are samples of body materials, such as blood, urine, stool, sputum, and tissue, and specimen collection is a vital role for the nursing assistant. Specimens are collected and tested to help make accurate diagnoses and to aid in treatment decisions.

. . . .

All specimens should be considered potentially hazardous or infectious. Standard precautions should be observed when handling specimens.

. . . .

It is important to use aseptic technique when collecting specimens to avoid contaminating them. Wash hands carefully before and after collecting specimens.

Nursing Assistant/Nurse Aide Flash Review

GENERAL PRINCIPLES OF SPECIMEN COLLECTION

Nursing assistants should follow these guidelines when collecting specimens:

• Be accurate and follow directions precisely.

• Collect the specimen at the prescribed time.

• Verify that it is the correct client; check the name, identification number, and other identifying data.

• Label each specimen correctly and clearly, and attach the label immediately to the specimen container.

• Check for:
  • correct client.
  • correct specimen.
  • correct time.
  • correct amount.
  • correct container.
  • correct laboratory slip.
  • correct method/procedure.
  • correct asepsis.
  • correct attitude.

• Help client become comfortable after specimen collection.

• Report and document that the specific specimen was collected, that it was sent to the laboratory, the time and date it was collected, how the client tolerated the procedure, and any unusual observations.

. . . .

Nursing Assistant/Nurse Aide Flash Review

ROUTINE URINE SAMPLE

. . . .

Urine is usually collected when a client is admitted to run routine tests. To obtain a routine urine sample:

- Gather equipment.

- Wash hands.

- Prepare labels.

- Provide privacy.

- Explain procedure.

- Put on gloves.

- Have client urinate in clean bedpan, urinal, or specimen cup.

- If using bedpan or urinal, empty urine into graduated container and measure, if client is on I&O; then pour some of the urine into the specimen container.

- Place lid on the container, and place label on the container.

- Clean the equipment.

- Remove gloves and wash hands.

. . . .

ROUTINE URINE SAMPLE FROM AN INFANT

. . . .

To obtain a routine urine sample from an infant:

- Gather equipment.
- Wash hands.
- Prepare labels.
- Provide privacy.
- Explain procedure to parents.
- Put on gloves.
- Take off diaper.
- Clean and dry the skin around the genital area.
- Apply the urine collector over entire genital area.
- Put diaper back on.
- Remove gloves and wash hands.
- Check infant every half hour to see if infant has voided into the urine collector.
- Once infant has voided, wash hands, put gloves on, and carefully remove the collector.
- Wash off infant's genital area and replace diaper.
- Place urine in specimen container and cover container.
- Label the container.
- Take off gloves and wash hands.

Nursing Assistant/Nurse Aide Flash Review

CLEAN CATCH URINE SPECIMEN

PART
5

Clean catch urine samples must be obtained in a contamination-free manner. To do this, a special container must be used, the genital area must be cleaned, and the urine must be collected midstream. To obtain a clean catch urine specimen:

- Gather equipment, including a clean catch urine kit.
- Wash hands.
- Prepare labels.
- Provide privacy.
- Explain procedure and allow client to collect own specimen if able, using the cleaning procedure.
- Put on gloves and open the kit.
- For female clients:
    - Use all three towelettes from the clean catch kit.
    - Separate the labia and wipe one side from front to back with one towelette.
    - Wipe the other side from front to back with another towelette.
    - Wipe down the middle from front to back with the third towelette.
- For male clients:
    - If the client is not circumcised, pull back the foreskin for cleaning and hold it back during urination.
    - Clean the head of the penis using a circular motion and the towelettes.
- If client is able to start and stop stream, explain that he or she is to start urinating, stop, start again, and then collect specimen in the container. The client must remove container before stopping urinating.
- If client cannot start and stop urinating, the nursing assistant will collect the specimen midstream.
- Cover the container and label it.
- Clean permanent equipment and discard disposable equipment.
- Remove gloves and wash hands.

COLLECTING 24-HOUR URINE SPECIMEN

. . . .

REAGENT STRIPS

. . . .

PART 5

Sometimes physicians order 24-hour urine specimens to test for specific disease processes. For these specimens, the client discards the first morning void, then begins the test and collects all urine in a special container for 24 hours. If any urine is lost, the test must start again.

· ·

Sometimes reagent (dip) sticks are used to test urine for sugar, pH, blood, specific gravity, ketones, and other materials. These tests can be done quickly, and thus, they are often used for rapid diagnosis and treatment. Reagent strips vary, but most should be stored at room temperature and out of direct sunlight.

· ·

STOOL SPECIMENS

Stool specimens can also help diagnose certain conditions, including parasites. However, most stool specimens must be collected and submitted while they are still fresh and warm. To collect a stool specimen:

- Gather equipment, including a clean catch urine kit.

- Wash hands.

- Prepare labels.

- Provide privacy.

- Explain procedure and allow client to collect own specimen if able, using the cleaning procedure.

- Put on gloves.

- If the client uses a toilet or commode, fit the specimen collection device underneath the toilet or commode seat. If not, provide the client with a bedpan.

- Remind client not to urinate, and make sure client has toilet paper and a container in which to dispose of it.

- Have client signal when he or she is finished stooling.

- Once client signals, return, wash hands, and put on gloves.

- Assist client with hand washing, and help client return to bed if he or she used toilet or commode.

- Remove bedpan, cover it, and provide for perineal care and hand washing if client used bedpan.

- Bring bedpan or collection device to the bathroom.

- Observe color, consistency, or amount of stool.

- Use a tongue depressor to collect about two tablespoons of stool and place it in the specimen container; cover the container with the lid.

- Place container on paper towel on counter.

- Label the container.

- Remove one glove, hold the transport bag with that ungloved hand, and place the labeled container in the transport bag with the gloved hand. Do not touch the outside of the bag with the gloved hand or container.

- Remove other glove and wash hands.

Nursing Assistant/Nurse Aide Flash Review

STOOL SPECIMEN FOR BLOOD

. . . .

SPUTUM SPECIMEN

. . . .

Nursing assistants may be asked to collect stool and set it on a Hemoccult® slide so that the stool can be tested for blood.

· ·

Sputum consists of mucous and other materials coughed up from the respiratory tract. When collecting sputum:

- Gather equipment, including a clean catch urine kit.

- Wash hands.

- Prepare labels.

- Provide privacy.

- Explain procedure and allow client to collect own specimen if able, using the cleaning procedure.

- Put on gloves.

- Have client rinse mouth with mouthwash before coughing.

- Ask client to cough and spit into sterile specimen cup.

- Close lid on cup and label it.

- Remove gloves and wash hands.

· ·

ALTERNATIVES TO RESTRAINTS

. . . .

PURPOSE OF RESTRAINTS

. . . .

WHEN RESTRAINTS ARE NOT USED

PART
5

Restraint-free care has gained popularity thanks to government agencies and advocacy groups. Alternatives to restraints include finding and correcting the underlying problem, such as pain and chemical imbalance, or the stressor that led to violent or self-destructive behavior; other alternatives are providing food and beverages, offering relaxation techniques, frequently reorienting client when client is confused, individualizing client care, eliminating tubes and drains or making them less obvious to clients, distraction, family involvement, moving client closer to the nursing station, and providing the client with familiar items. Wandering clients may be fitted with a wandering monitor sensor that sets off an alarm if they try to leave the facility.

. . . .

Restraints may be chemical (medication) or physical (mitts, soft restraints, leather restraints). Restraints are used to limit movement or access to one's body to prevent that person from hurting self or others or from removing necessary medical devices. Restraints may also be used to prevent a person from wandering from a facility due to dementia. Nurses and other staff first use other alternatives to keep client and others safe; however, physical restraints are necessary at times. The Joint Commission discourages their use altogether. OBRA notes that these devices should be used only when a client may hurt self or others or to protect a client during a medical procedure, and only with a physician's order. Physical restraints are, thus, used as protective devices when other methods have failed and only with a physician's order.

. . . .

Restraints should never be used for staff convenience or as a punishment to the client.

TYPES OF PHYSICAL RESTRAINTS

· ·

COMPLICATIONS OF RESTRAINTS

· ·

PART 5

RESTRAINT POLICIES

- Mitts are padded covers placed over the hands to prevent the client from grabbing things like IV tubing.

- Soft limb restraints are typically made from cloth and used on the limbs for short-term cases such as postsurgical agitation.

- Leather restraints are reserved for extreme emergencies when the client is a danger to self or others. They are usually used for clients who are violent, under the influence of mood-altering drugs, or very confused.

- Lap buddies and chair trays are considered restraints if the client cannot remove the device independently.

· ·

Complications of restraints include:

- stress

- negative impact on cognitive skills

- increased confusion

- increased agitation

- injuries (abrasions, bruises, fractures, nerve damage)

- pressure ulcers

- pneumonia

- deep vein thrombosis

- death by strangulation or asphyxia

· ·

Restraint orders must include the type of restraint to be used and justification for same. As needed (prn) restraint orders are not permitted. Facilities have their own restraint policies, but most include 24-hour written order follow-up to verbal orders, face-to-face physician examination of the client every day or shift, vigilant monitoring and documentation, and the removal of the restraints at the earliest possible time.

APPLYING RESTRAINTS

. . . .

CARE OF CLIENTS IN RESTRAINTS

. . . .

WRIST AND ANKLE RESTRAINTS

PART 5

Most facilities require that nurses apply restraints. However, nursing assistants will provide care for clients who are in restraints.

. . . .

When using restraints:

- Ensure that there is a physician's order.
- Use the least restrictive device for the shortest period of time.
- Follow directions/instructions for use.
- Use restraints that are in good condition and the correct size.
- Do not create and use makeshift restraints.
- Knots should be tied in a quick release manner.
- Have adequate help when applying restraints.
- Check the person every 15 minutes and ensure that sensation and blood flow are not impaired.
- Make sure wheels on beds and wheelchairs are locked.
- Make sure side rails are up.
- Remove restraints every two hours for 10 minutes.
- Report and document.

. . . .

Wrist and ankle restraints are used to prevent clients from moving these limbs. They may be used to keep a client in bed, but are usually used to keep the client from removing medical devices.

. . . .

BELT RESTRAINT

. . . .

VEST RESTRAINT

. . . .

PART
5

A belt restraint, also called lap or waist restraint, is used to prevent clients from sliding out of chairs, but can also be used to prevent clients from sliding out of bed.

· ·

A vest restraint is used to prevent clients from falling out of the bed or chair. They should never be put on backward (flaps across the back and back of vest across the chest), because the client can strangle to death if he or she slides down against it.

· ·

Nursing Assistant Care of Special Populations

CHANGES DURING PREGNANCY

. . . .

A woman's body undergoes transformations to accommodate the growth and development of the fetus. These changes come from hormones that are secreted by the pituitary gland and the placenta; the placenta develops from the lining of the uterus to provide and exchange gases and nutrients between the fetus and mother. The uterus enlarges to allow the fetus to grow; the breasts begin to develop milk, and more blood is created to allow for the deliverance of nutrients to the fetus and removal of waste products from the fetus. These changes can result in the signs and symptoms of pregnancy over each trimester:

- First trimester: loss of menstrual periods; swollen and tender breasts; possible morning sickness

- Second trimester: abdominal enlargement from enlarged uterus; weight gain; enlarged breasts; feeling the fetus move

- Third trimester: shortness of breath and indigestion from enlarged uterus pressing on organs; possible trouble sleeping; swollen ankles

Nursing Assistant/Nurse Aide Flash Review

COMPLICATIONS OF PREGNANCY

. . . .

PRENATAL CARE

. . . .

PART 6

Some women experience complications during their pregnancies. These include:

- preterm labor when labor begins before fetus can survive on its own
- preeclampsia or eclampsia when the mother develops severe hypertension
- anemia from inadequate healthy red blood cells
- depression during or after pregnancy
- ectopic pregnancy when the fertilized egg implants outside the uterus
- gestational diabetes when the blood sugar is high during pregnancy
- miscarriage when the mother loses the pregnancy before 20 weeks from natural causes
- fetal problems when any number of problems can affect the fetus or newborn

Some mothers are at risk before pregnancy due to preexisting health problems. When prenatal health issues are severe and cause risk to the mother or fetus, the mother may be hospitalized for more intensive care. If working with a hospitalized pregnant mother, the nursing assistant should document and report:

- changes in vital signs
- complaints of headaches or visual disturbances
- fainting or dizziness
- nausea, vomiting, or diarrhea
- abdominal pain
- uterine contractions
- vaginal bleeding or discharge

. . . .

Prenatal care decreases the risk of complications by helping to ensure the health of the mother and fetus. Prenatal care should begin when a woman believes she is pregnant.

. . . .

LABOR AND DELIVERY

. . . .

Labor is the process by which uterine contractions squeeze the infant downward, pushing his or her head against the cervix and forcing it to dilate. The time of labor varies greatly. Mothers may deliver vaginally (baby born through the vagina) or by cesarean section (baby is delivered through a surgical opening in the mother's abdomen and uterus). The latter is performed when there are certain complications, including long-term labor and incorrect position of the baby.

While women who deliver vaginally may choose not to have some form of anesthesia, those who deliver by cesarean section need anesthesia because this is a surgical procedure. Anesthesia may be general or an epidural block, which is given by catheter into the spinal canal and affects only the lower body. The nursing assistant's role in labor and delivery is usually very limited, unless the nursing assistant works in a birthing center and receives additional education.

• •

Nursing Assistant/Nurse Aide Flash Review

POSTPARTUM CARE

. . . .

Nursing assistants may care for mothers after delivery. Postpartum care includes:

- monitoring vital signs
- assisting with mobility
- assisting with toileting
- assisting with breast-feeding
- monitoring and managing vaginal discharge, called lochia:
  - Rubra lochia is bright red and will exist for two or three days.
  - Lochia serosa follows and is a pink- or brown-tinged fluid that lasts for 3 to 10 days; large clots should be reported right away.
  - Lochia alba is last and is a creamy white or yellow discharge that lasts an additional one or two weeks.
- Observing for complications, which should be immediately reported:
  - increased vaginal bleeding
  - foul-smelling vaginal discharge or drainage from a cesarean incision
  - breast pain or swelling
  - changes in vital signs
  - pain that increases or persists after medication
  - dizziness
  - excessive thirst
  - chest pain or trouble breathing
  - trouble voiding
  - increased numbness in legs after an epidural block
  - signs of depression or sadness

NEWBORN CARE

. . . .

SIGNS OF ILL NEWBORN

. . . .

Nursing assistants may care for newborns in the hospital, in a birthing center, or during home care. Newborn care includes:

- monitoring vital signs
- ensuring security
- feeding if the infant is not breast-fed
- burping
- changing diapers using standard precautions
- bathing
- assisting with sleep (babies should be placed on their back or side without blankets, other fluffy bedding, pillows, or toys to prevent suffocation)
- transporting (all states require that the infant be placed correctly in a car seat, which is installed into the backseat of the car, facing backward)
- caring for the umbilical cord
- providing circumcision care
- following abduction-prevention policies to prevent child from being abducted

. . . .

Newborns can become very sick quickly. Report the following immediately to the nurse:

- weakness or floppiness
- pale color
- discolored eyes (e.g., red or yellow sclera)
- inconsolable crying
- inability to wake baby
- high or low temperature
- abnormal heart rate
- rapid, shallow breathing
- rash
- not feeding
- vomiting

. . . .

FAMILY

· ·

INFANT CARE

· ·

TODDLER CARE

PART
6

Family involvement, especially parental involvement, is critical in pediatric care. The family provides support for the pediatric client, and this support promotes healing. Parents also need to feel that they are not giving up their parenting role, and thus, should be encouraged to care for their child as much as possible.

. . . .

Infants are completely dependent on adults. When caring for infants, nursing assistants will monitor vital signs, as well as food and fluid intake, and feed, diaper, bathe, and position the infant. Infants need to feel secure through human contact such as holding, touching, and rocking. Accident prevention is also important:

- Do not leave infant unattended on a surface where the infant can roll off, or in any amount of water.
- Use straps when infant is in high chair or carrier.
- Remove all small items to prevent choking.
- Remove all plastic bags and balloons to prevent suffocation.
- Keep infant away from cords that can cause strangulation.

. . . .

Toddlers are mobile and curious, and safety measures should include the prevention of falls, wandering, drowning, and poisoning. They are also independent and may not cooperate at times.

Toddlers may also experience separation anxiety when parents leave or regression from the stress of hospitalization, returning to an earlier stage of development. If this happens, the previously toilet-trained toddler may soil.

PRESCHOOLER CARE

. . . .

SCHOOL-AGE CHILD CARE

. . . .

ADOLESCENT CARE

PART
6

[465]

Preschoolers have most of their self-help skills, such as toileting and brushing their teeth, although some regress when ill. Preschoolers also have magical thinking and think that if they wish something, it will happen. This also causes them to believe that they are being punished when they are ill and under treatment, and thus, they need reassurance. Preschoolers need simple answers to their questions, as well as simple explanations of procedures. Using their dolls or stuffed animals helps them to understand what is expected.

• •

School-age children have a sense of right and wrong and like to learn. They want their questions answered and appreciate rewards. School-age children need peer support, so phone calls, e-mails, cards, and visits are helpful for their recovery.

• •

Adolescents can do their own care and usually do not like being dependent on others. Privacy is critical, and most are concerned about body image, which can be diminished by illness. This is a period of intense growth, and thus, most need extra snacks between meals. Peanut butter, cheese, crackers, and fruits are healthy and teen-appropriate foods. Many adolescents are admitted due to mental illness or accidents, and some teens also experience sexually transmitted diseases and pregnancy. These all require sensitivity on the part of the nursing assistant.

• •

CHILD ABUSE

. . . .

RISK FACTORS FOR CHILD ABUSE

. . . .

Like the elderly, children are vulnerable and thus, may be targets of abuse.

- Physical abuse is the intentional infliction of injury to a child by a caretaker that can result in bruising, burns, fractures, poisoning, and head or abdominal trauma.

- Emotional abuse is the deliberate attempt to destroy the child's self-esteem or competence by rejecting, ignoring, criticizing, isolating, or terrorizing the child.

- Neglect is the failure of the child's parent or legal guardian to provide a minimum degree of care in supplying the child with adequate food, clothing, shelter, or education or medical care.

- Sexual abuse is contact or interaction between a child and an adult when the child is used for sexual stimulation of an adult.

. . . .

Risk factors for child abuse include:

- Caretaker factors
    - severe punishment of caretakers themselves as children
    - poor impulse control
    - free expression of violence
    - social isolation
    - poor social-emotional support system
    - substance abuse

- Child factors
    - illness, disability, and developmental delay
    - illegitimate or unwanted pregnancy
    - hyperkinesis
    - bonding failure
    - problem pregnancy, delivery, or prematurity

- Environmental factors (all socioeconomic groups are affected)
    - chronic stress
    - poverty, poor housing, unemployment
    - divorce
    - frequent relocation

. . . .

Nursing Assistant/Nurse Aide Flash Review

SIGNS OF CHILD ABUSE

....

NURSING ASSISTANT'S ROLE IN CHILD ABUSE

....

- Child has unexplained burns, bites, bruises, broken bones, or black eyes.
- Child seems frightened of the parents and protests or cries when it is time to go home.
- Child reports injury by a parent or another adult caregiver.
- Caretakers offer conflicting, unconvincing, or no explanation for the child's injury.
- Child lacks needed medical or dental care, immunizations, or glasses.
- Consistently dirty and has severe body odor.
- States that there is no one at home to provide care.
- Has difficulty walking or sitting.
- Reports nightmares or bedwetting.
- Experiences a sudden change in appetite.
- Demonstrates bizarre, sophisticated, or unusual sexual knowledge or behavior.
- Becomes pregnant or contracts a venereal disease, particularly if under age 14.
- Runs away.
- Reports sexual abuse by a parent or another adult caregiver.
- Shows extremes in behavior, such as overly compliant or demanding behavior, extreme passivity, or aggression.
- Acts either inappropriately adult (parenting other children, for example) or inappropriately infantile (frequently rocking or head-banging, for example).

. . . .

Nursing assistants should be observant for signs of child abuse and should report these signs and their suspicions to the nurse or their supervisor. They also are responsible for meeting the physical and emotional needs of the children in their care.

. . . .

TYPES OF SURGERY

. . . .

TYPES OF ANESTHESIA

. . . .

Surgery involves entering the body to physically remove or repair damaged organs and tissue. Types of surgery include:

- Exploratory: problem exists, but there is uncertainty as to what it is.
- Definitive surgery: surgical intervention for a known problem.
- Elective: surgery is planned for ahead of time.
- Urgent: surgery is planned for as soon as possible.
- Emergent: surgery must be performed immediately to avoid severe consequences.

Most surgeries have three stages: preoperative stage before surgery, the intraoperative stage during surgery, and the postoperative stage after surgery.

. . . .

Most surgeries require some type of anesthesia to prevent the person from feeling pain during the procedure. Types are:

- General anesthesia creates a full loss of consciousness.
- Regional anesthesia causes loss of sensation in one part of the body but the person remains conscious.
- Local anesthesia causes loss of sensation in a small area and the person remains conscious.

. . . .

PREOPERATIVE CARE

. . . .

INTRAOPERATIVE CARE

. . . .

PART 6

Preoperative care begins when the client is informed about the surgery. This can last for several weeks for elective surgeries and minutes for emergent ones. During this phase, the person is prepared emotionally and physically. Preliminary diagnostic/baseline tests are performed, and informed consent is obtained. The client is NPO for six to eight hours prior to surgery to prevent aspiration of vomitus. Nursing assistants help clients the morning of surgery by assisting with morning care, assuring that makeup, nail polish, jewelry, glasses, contact lenses, prosthetic devices, and other items are removed prior to surgery, and that the client puts on a hospital gown. Some clients also require site preparation (cleansing and shaving) or enemas before surgery.

. . . .

The nursing assistant usually prepares the client's room while the client is undergoing surgery. This includes:

- changing the bed linens and making a surgical bed

- raising the bed to allow for client transfer from the operating room stretcher

- moving furniture if needed to clear a path for the stretcher

- gathering necessary items: vital signs equipment, flow sheets, IV pole, emesis basin, linen/bed protector, suction equipment, extra pillows or positioning aids, and warm blankets

. . . .

POSTOPERATIVE CARE

. . . .

PREVENTING POSTOPERATIVE COMPLICATIONS

. . . .

PART 6

Most surgical clients are taken to the postanesthesia care unit (PACU) or recovery room immediately after surgery. Here the client is closely monitored to help the client recover without complications. Once the client awakens and is oriented and stable, the client is brought back to the unit.

When the client returns to the unit, the nursing assistant helps with transferring the client from the stretcher to the bed. While the nurse will assess the client's condition, the nursing assistant may take the client's vital signs and may continue to do this every 15 minutes for the first hour, every 30 minutes for the next hour or two, and then every four hours thereafter, unless otherwise ordered. The nursing assistant will also help with preventing complications and assisting with positioning, nutrition, elimination, hygiene, pain control, and ambulation.

· ·

Postoperative clients are at risk for complications, especially cardiac and respiratory complications. Respiratory complications include pneumonia and atelectasis (collapse of alveoli). To help prevent these complications, nursing assistants may aid client with coughing and deep-breathing exercises and incentive spirometry, where the person forcefully exhales into an incentive spirometer. Cardiac problems include the development of blood clots. These can be prevented with the use of antiembolism stockings, leg exercises, and a sequential compression device (SCD) that helps prevent pooling of blood in the calves.

· ·

NURSING ASSISTANT REPORTING OF POSTOPERATIVE COMPLICATIONS

When caring for clients in the postoperative period, nursing assistants should report:

- restlessness or confusion
- increased complaints of pain
- pain, numbness, or tingling at cast site
- increased bleeding at dressing site
- changes in vital signs
- respiratory problems
- pale or blue lips or nail beds
- cool and clammy skin

. . . .

Nursing Assistant/Nurse Aide Flash Review

DEFINITION OF MENTAL HEALTH

. . . .

PSYCHIATRIST

. . . .

PSYCHOLOGIST

PART
6

Mental health is a state of emotional balance and the absence of mental illness.

. . . .

A psychiatrist is a medical physician who diagnoses and treats mental illness.

. . . .

A psychologist is an educated professional who provides counseling services, and who also diagnoses and treats mental illnesses, but usually is not allowed by law to prescribe medications.

STRESS

. . . .

POTENTIAL FOR SELF-HARM

. . . .

PART
6

Everyone experiences stress, especially developmental stressors (adolescence, midlife) and situation stressors (moving, new job). Some people also experience catastrophic stressors, such as war, natural disasters, and violent crime victimization. Everyone deals with stress differently, and people can handle different amounts of stress at different times in their lives. Multiple or cumulative stressors can bring a person to the breaking point, causing someone to have trouble eating, sleeping, and/or concentrating.

People manage stress with defense mechanisms such as denial and rationalization, and coping mechanisms that include prayer, exercise, and hobbies.

• •

People with mental illness are at increased risk for suicide. Diagnosis and treatment of mental illness is critical.

• •

Nursing Assistant/Nurse Aide Flash Review

CLIENTS WITH ANXIETY DISORDERS

. . . .

CLIENTS WITH AFFECTIVE DISORDERS

. . . .

PART
6

Anxiety is a normal feeling of uneasiness and worry. However, some people experience anxiety to a degree where it interferes with their activities of daily living:

- Phobia means an excessive fear of a specific object (snakes, spiders) or situation (public speaking, flying). The person may go to extremes to avoid the fear. Some people avoid leaving the house altogether; they have developed agoraphobia, a fear of open or public places.

- Panic disorder creates sudden overpowering fear to the point of panic attacks. During these attacks, the person experiences physical symptoms like chest pain that can mimic a heart attack. While not physiological, the symptoms are real.

- Obsessive-compulsive disorder causes people to suffer from recurrent intrusive thoughts or obsessions (being surrounded by germs) and behaviors or compulsions (washing hands frequently). Their ritualistic behavior interferes with their quality of life, but not doing it creates extreme anxiety.

- Posttraumatic stress disorder (PTSD) occurs after a traumatic event (war, assault, disaster). The person experiences flashbacks (memories of the event so real they feel they are reliving it), panic attacks, and depression. PTSD is seen in soldiers returning from war.

. . . .

Affective disorders are also called mood disorders.

- Depression is marked by feelings of sadness and hopelessness. The person may also lose interest in pleasurable activities, have trouble sleeping, eat too much or too little, and have feelings of guilt. Some persons with depression are irritable and restless.

- Bipolar disorder, also known as manic-depression, is characterized by periods of depression and mania. Mania can result in impulsive and reckless behaviors.

. . . .

CLIENTS WITH SCHIZOPHRENIA

. . . .

CLIENTS WITH SUBSTANCE ABUSE

. . . .

PART
6

Schizophrenia is a disabling mental illness that is characterized by psychosis (break with reality). The person experiences hallucinations (faulty sensory perceptions, especially visual and auditory hallucinations) and/or delusions (faulty ideas, such as believing one is being chased by the CIA). Persons with schizophrenia also have problems with thinking, speech, and behaviors.

. . . .

Substance abuse disorders involve the abuse of alcohol; drugs (illegal, prescription, or over-the-counter); or inhalants (glue). Addiction is the physical need for the drug, and withdrawal is the reaction that happens when the substance is suddenly taken away. Withdrawal can be an emergency; the nursing assistant should report:

- changes in mental status or mood

- restlessness

- anxiety or fear

- delirium

- hallucinations (usually tactile, feeling as though something is crawling on the skin)

- insomnia

- tremors

- sweating

- nausea and vomiting

- rapid pulse or palpitations

- seizures

. . . .

CLIENTS WITH EATING DISORDERS

. . . .

CARING FOR CLIENTS WITH MENTAL ILLNESS

. . . .

PART 6

Eating disorders involve abnormal eating patterns and a preoccupation with thinness. These are serious problems that can lead to suicide, kidney failure, and death.

- Anorexia nervosa has been described as the relentless pursuit of thinness. Those with this disorder see themselves as fat, despite being very thin. They also eat very little and exercise frequently.

- Bulimia nervosa is characterized by binge eating and mechanisms to avoid weight gain, such as self-induced vomiting or the use of laxatives, both considered purging. These persons are also very concerned about their weight.

. . . .

Nursing assistants frequently care for clients with mental illness who are admitted to hospitals and long-term care facilities, as well as psychiatric hospitals. Nursing assistants can use their observation, listening, and communication skills to note subtle changes and help ensure that clients receive prompt treatment. The nursing assistant should report:

- changes in eating, sleeping, and/or activity patterns
- restlessness
- inability to concentrate
- prolonged crying
- loss of interest in previously enjoyed activities
- loss of interest in socializing with others
- unusual mood changes
- unusual behavioral changes
- hopelessness
- giving away personal possessions
- talking about wanting to die

. . . .

Nursing Assistant/Nurse Aide Flash Review

HIV/AIDS

. . . .

HIV/AIDS SYMPTOMS

. . . .

PART 6

Acquired immunodeficiency syndrome (AIDS) is a potentially life-threatening illness caused by the human immunodeficiency virus (HIV). It damages the immune system, reducing the body's ability to fight infection.

. . . .

- fever
- weight loss
- fatigue
- muscle soreness
- rash
- headache
- sore throat
- difficulty swallowing
- mouth or genital ulcers
- swollen lymph glands, mainly on the neck
- joint pain
- night sweats
- diarrhea
- confusion

. . . .

Nursing Assistant/Nurse Aide Flash Review

RISK FACTORS FOR HIV/AIDS

. . . .

RIGHTS OF PERSON WITH HIV/AIDS

. . . .

CARE OF CLIENTS WITH HIV/AIDS

PART 6

- unprotected sex, anal sex, and sex with multiple partners
- using intravenous drugs and sharing dirty needles
- having another sexually transmitted disease with open sores that act as gateway for HIV
- blood products or transfusions (a rare risk after 1985, but possible in developing countries where blood supplies are not screened)

. . . .

Some cultures still view HIV/AIDS as shameful, creating fear and discrimination. Because of discrimination, many states have laws that protect the rights of persons with HIV/AIDS regarding their education, employment, privacy, and health care. Nursing assistants are responsible for maintaining strict confidentiality of clients' HIV/AIDS status.

. . . .

The level of care depends on the extent of the client's illness. Care may include:

- mouth care for sores that develop in the mouth
- promotion of adequate nutrition because of mouth sores and lack of appetite
- maintenance of hydration because of chronic diarrhea
- monitoring of intake and output (I&O)
- skin care for rashes
- infection control due to poor immune status
- emotional support

DEVELOPMENTAL DISABILITY

. . . .

MENTAL RETARDATION (INTELLECTUAL DISABILITY)

. . . .

AUTISTIC SPECTRUM DISORDERS

PART 6

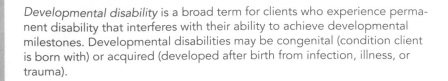

Developmental disability is a broad term for clients who experience permanent disability that interferes with their ability to achieve developmental milestones. Developmental disabilities may be congenital (condition client is born with) or acquired (developed after birth from infection, illness, or trauma).

· ·

Intellectual disability is the combination of an intelligence quotient (IQ) below 70 (thinking, reasoning, understanding difficulties) and problems with adaptive functioning (ability to carry out activities of daily living [ADLs]).

- Mild intellectual disability: Person achieves abilities of a third to sixth grade level. This is the most common type of intellectual disability and may go unnoticed until the child has difficulties in school.

- Moderate intellectual disability: Person achieves up to a second grade level and has delays in speech and motor skills. The person may have difficulty with socially appropriate behavior.

- Severe intellectual disability: Person can learn some communication and basic skills.

- Profound intellectual disability: Person has minimal functioning in all developmental areas and needs constant assistance and supervision.

· ·

Autistic spectrum disorders cover the wide spectrum of autism. People with autism have difficulty with communicating and relating to others. They may also have problems with their ability to perform ADLs and their response to touch and pain.

Nursing Assistant/Nurse Aide Flash Review

DOWN SYNDROME

. . . .

CEREBRAL PALSY

. . . .

FETAL ALCOHOL SYNDROME

PART
6

Down syndrome is a genetic disorder that usually causes mild to moderate mental retardation. Some cases may be severe, whereas others have normal intelligence. The features of Down syndrome include flattened facial features, small head, short neck, protruding tongue, upward-slanting eyes, and unusually shaped ears. Complications include heart disease, obesity, leukemia, dementia, and sleep apnea. Many people with Down syndrome live independently and hold jobs. Most live with their families, whereas others live in group homes.

. . . .

Cerebral palsy (CP) is a broad term for a group of disorders that impair movement control due to damage to the developing brain. CP is nonprogressive, meaning the brain damage does not continue to worsen throughout life. However, the symptoms due to the brain damage can change over time, sometimes getting better and sometimes getting worse. There are different types of CP. One type causes spasms and another causes involuntary movements. Some people with CP have an intellectual disability, whereas others have normal intelligence.

. . . .

Fetal alcohol syndrome (FAS) results from alcohol exposure during pregnancy. Problems vary from child to child, but characteristics include physical deformities, mental retardation, learning disorders, vision difficulties, and behavioral problems. No amount of alcohol is known to be safe to consume during pregnancy.

SPINA BIFIDA

....

HEALTHCARE SETTINGS FOR PERSONS WITH DISABILITIES

....

ABUSE

PART
6

Spina bifida is a group of birth defects called neural tube defects. The neural tube is the embryonic structure that develops into the baby's brain and spinal cord. In babies with spina bifida, a portion of the neural tube does not develop properly, causing defects in the spinal cord and in the spine. Spina bifida occurs in various forms of severity. Some children have a barely visible deformity and no complications, while others are born with an open sack of spinal nerves that causes severe problems such as paralysis and poor bladder and bowel control.

. . . .

Persons with disabilities may be cared for by their families, as well as by:

- hospitals
- home health agencies
- day care centers
- long-term care facilities

. . . .

Persons with disabilities are at increased risk for abuse.

CARING FOR A PERSON WITH DEVELOPMENTAL DISABILITY

....

Caring for a person with developmental disability includes assisting with communication and activities of daily living. When caring for a client with a developmental disability, report:

- changes in vital signs
- changes in appetite, activity level, sleep patterns, or physical abilities
- change in mental status
- change in behavior
- signs of abuse

DEMENTIA

. . . .

SIGNS OF DEMENTIA

. . . .

TYPES

PART
6

Dementia describes a group of symptoms that affect thinking and social abilities severely enough to interfere with daily functioning. Dementia is permanent and progressive.

. . . .

- memory loss, especially short-term memory
- communication problems
- judgment problems
- disorientation
- inability to manage ADLs

. . . .

There are multiple types of dementia, but the most common cause is Alzheimer's disease:

- Alzheimer's disease is a slowly progressive disease characterized by plaques in the brain. It usually develops after age 50, but there is also an early-onset form of this disorder.

- Lewy body dementia is similar to Alzheimer's disease. Some persons develop Lewy bodies (clumps of protein) in the brain. Characteristics include fluctuations between confusion and clear thinking (lucidity), visual hallucinations, and tremors and rigidity (parkinsonism).

- Vascular dementia results from brain damage due to reduced or blocked blood flow in blood vessels leading to the brain. Symptoms usually start suddenly, and are more common in persons with high blood pressure or who have had strokes or heart attacks in the past.

- Frontotemporal dementia is less common but tends to occur at a younger age than does Alzheimer's disease, usually between the ages of 40 and 65. This is characterized by the breakdown of nerve cells in the frontal and temporal lobes of the brain that generally are associated with personality, behavior, and language.

Nursing Assistant/Nurse Aide Flash Review

RISK FACTORS OF DEMENTIA

. . . .

STAGES

. . . .

SYMPTOMS OF DEMENTIA

PART 6

Risk factors of dementia are advanced age, family history of dementia, Down syndrome, alcohol use, atherosclerosis, high blood pressure, high cholesterol, depression, diabetes, smoking, and obesity.

. . . .

Dementia can last for years. The three stages are:

1. Early: Memory loss begins. The person is aware of this, which causes anxiety, fear, depression, and/or anger.

2. Middle: The person begins to have difficulty communicating and recognizing familiar things and people, personality changes, and incontinence.

3. Late: The person loses the ability to sit and walk, is no longer able to speak, and becomes totally incontinent. Death follows.

. . . .

Dementia symptoms vary, but common ones include memory loss, difficulty communicating, difficulty with complex tasks, difficulty with planning and organizing, difficulty with coordination and motor functions, problems with disorientation such as wandering, personality changes, inability to reason, inappropriate behavior, paranoia, agitation, and hallucinations.

WANDERING

. . . .

PACING

. . . .

REPETITION

PART 6

People with dementia may wander. This is dangerous and can result in serious harm since the person can wander out into the cold and develop hypothermia or can drown. Since this is common, many long-term care facilities manage this by creating safe spaces for wandering, such as courtyards. Others use alert systems and attach sensors to the elder's ankle to set off an alarm if the person wanders.

. . . .

Continuous pacing may be due to an unmet need, such as hunger, fear, or overstimulation. Other times the person just needs to pace. If a need cannot be met, allow the person to pace safely.

. . . .

Saying or doing the same thing over and over again is called perseveration. These behaviors are not harmful, but may be managed with distraction if they annoy other clients.

RUMMAGING

. . . .

DELUSIONS AND HALLUCINATIONS

. . . .

AGITATION

Persons with dementia may rummage through closets or drawers. This may be managed by locking away other clients' items and helping clients with dementia to find what they are looking for.

. . . .

Delusions (faulty ideas) and hallucinations (faulty sensory perceptions) are common in persons with dementia. But unlike other disorders, it is best to go along with them and reassure these clients, as well as redirect them.

. . . .

Agitation is common, and clients may shout or strike at caregivers and other clients. This can be due to communication difficulties, pain, or unmet needs. To manage agitation and aggressive behavior:

- Talk in a calm voice.
- Remove client from the area and to a quiet environment.
- Document the possible causes of agitation and remove them in the future, when possible.
- Be consistent.
- Make sure client has hearing aids and glasses if needed.

Nursing Assistant/Nurse Aide Flash Review

CATASTROPHIC REACTIONS

. . . .

SUNDOWNING

. . . .

INAPPROPRIATE SEXUAL BEHAVIORS

PART
6

Clients with dementia may overreact to situations, especially when feeling threatened. These reactions may be minimized by approaching the client from the front, not rushing, knowing the client's preferences, and avoiding overfatigue and sudden changes in routine.

. . . .

Clients with dementia tend to worsen in late afternoon or evening. The cause is unknown but may be due to fatigue or visual difficulties. Interventions include providing care early in the day, creating a calm environment after sundown, offering fluids, turning on lights before dark, and providing clues such as clocks and calendars. Establishing a nighttime routine may also be beneficial.

. . . .

Clients may masturbate in public or climb into bed with another client. These clients must be redirected because staff has a responsibility to protect the other clients from unwanted sexual advances.

Nursing Assistant/Nurse Aide Flash Review

CARING FOR CLIENT WITH DEMENTIA

. . . .

CARING FOR CLIENT IN LATE STAGE OF DEMENTIA

. . . .

CAREGIVER STRESS

PART 6

When caring for a person with dementia:

- Maintain a structured and quiet environment.
- Assist client with bathing, dressing, eating, elimination, and ambulation.
- Avoid arguing.
- Use short words and phrases.
- Give the client time to respond.
- Listen carefully and observe nonverbal cues.
- Help client feel secure.
- Help client maintain independence for as long as possible.
- Encourage mind exercises.
- Protect client from injuries.
- Maintain client's personal hygiene.
- Take time out if frustration sets in.

. . . .

Clients become completely dependent in the late stage, and they are at risk for the complications of immobility. Once a client stops eating, death is imminent. This is a difficult time for the family, who may need to make decisions about advance directives.

. . . .

Caring for a loved one with dementia is difficult. Family members need support, understanding, and encouragement. They may also need respite care that allows for someone else to care for their loved one while they get some rest.

STAGES OF GRIEF

. . . .

ADVANCE DIRECTIVES

. . . .

HOSPICE CARE

PART
6

There are five stages of grief. However, people do not necessarily go through them in order, nor do all people go through all of them.

1. Denial, numbness, and shock: This stage protects the client from the impact of the loss, but it can be misinterpreted as being uncaring.

2. Bargaining: This stage of grief may be marked by persistent thoughts about what could have been done to prevent the loss or what one would give up to reverse it.

3. Depression: During this stage the client feels the full impact of the loss and exhibits signs of depression.

4. Anger: The person feels helpless and powerless, as well as angry due to abandonment because of the death.

5. Acceptance: The person comes to terms with all the emotions and feelings that were experienced when the death occurred. Healing can begin as the loss becomes integrated into the person's set of life experiences.

. . . .

Advance directives are legal documents that allow clients to detail their decisions about end-of-life care ahead of time. They tell the client's wishes to family, friends, and healthcare professionals to avoid confusion later on. The person can make decisions on the use of feeding tubes, resuscitation, and dialysis, as well as whether to donate organs and tissues.

. . . .

Hospice care is end-of-life care with medical, psychological, and spiritual support. The goal is to help people who are dying have peace, comfort, and dignity. Hospice programs can be at home, in a hospital, at a hospice, or in a skilled nursing facility. They also provide services to support a patient's family.

CARE OF THE DYING CLIENT

. . . .

CARE OF THE FAMILY

. . . .

PART
6

The dying client becomes increasingly dependent on others as death approaches, and the goal of care focuses on comfort.

- Provide skin and mucous membrane care. At this point the eyes may need ointment at night.
- Position frequently.
- Provide back rubs, soft music, or reading to make the person comfortable.
- Suctioning and oxygen therapy can make breathing easier.
- Keep the room well lit, and announce presence to help offset visual difficulties.
- Allow family members to assist with care.
- Be a good listener.
- Assist client with cultural and religious needs.

. . . .

Family members need to cope with the approaching loss of their loved one, and they may react in unexpected ways. The nursing assistant should not take their behavior personally and can help them by:

- maintaining communication
- allowing them to participate in the client's care
- ensuring that their needs are met
- caring for the client without being intrusive to the family

. . . .

POSTMORTEM CARE

. . . .

PART

6

The client's body should be treated with respect.

- Obtain supplies and postmortem kit.

- Set bed at a comfortable working height and lock the wheels.

- Put on gloves.

- Place the body in the supine position and place a pillow under the person's head and shoulders. Undress the body and cover it with bath blanket.

- Close the eyes. If they do not close, notify the nurse before the family arrives.

- Replace the person's dentures and close the mouth. Use a chin strap if the jaw needs support.

- Remove jewelry and place in an envelope for the family. List each piece of jewelry as it is removed.

- Wash the body and comb the hair.

- If the family will view the body, dress it in a clean gown, and change linens if soiled. Cover with top sheet.

- Straighten the room and provide for the family's privacy.

- Apply shroud.

- Transfer the body from the bed to a stretcher for transport to the morgue, if appropriate.

- Report and document the time the body was transported and the location of the person's belongings.

• •

REHABILITATION

. . . .

RESTORATIVE CARE

. . . .

REHABILITATION NEEDS

PART
6

Rehabilitation is the process that helps restore the state of optimal health for ill, injured, and disabled persons. Rehabilitation can be a long process, and sometimes only minor gains are possible. Therefore, rehabilitation requires the client's acceptance of gaining small accomplishments. Types of rehabilitation include:

- physical (physical, occupational, and speech-language therapies)
- emotional rehabilitation (e.g., helping client with coping skills)
- vocational (helping client gain employment)

. . . .

Restorative care helps clients keep their current level of independence or regain a higher level.

. . . .

Rehabilitation usually focuses on specific situations and affected body systems, for example:

- integumentary: burns
- cardiovascular: following heart attack or heart surgery
- neurological: strokes, traumatic brain injuries
- musculoskeletal: following joint replacement surgery, traumatic injuries
- digestive/urinary: bowel or bladder training
- endocrine: diabetes mellitus

OBRA REQUIREMENTS

. . . .

PHASES OF REHABILITATION

. . . .

REHABILITATION TEAM

PART 6

OBRA requires that clients receive the therapy outlined in their care plans.

. . . .

The three phases of rehabilitation are:

1. Acute: Clients require constant observation and care in the first 24 hours after injury, surgery, or serious illness. The goals at this time are to keep the client alive.

2. Subacute: This phase lasts about one week with the goal of stabilizing the client's condition and preventing the complications of immobility.

3. Chronic phase: In this phase, active rehabilitation and restorative care begin and continue. This may include restoring and maintaining the client's ability to perform ADLs, communicate, problem solve, and achieve financial independence.

. . . .

The rehabilitation team includes:

- Physiatrist is the physician who directs client care.

- Rehabilitation nurse provides direct care and teaching.

- Physical therapist helps client regain and maintain strength, endurance, and flexibility.

- Occupational therapist helps person with ADLs.

- Speech-language pathologist helps client regain and maintain communication, chewing, and swallowing skills.

- Neuropsychologist helps person regain and maintain cognitive skills.

- Orthotist fits clients for supportive devices, such as braces.

- Prosthesist fits clients for prosthetic devices, such as artificial limbs.

- Recreation therapist promotes client socialization and self-esteem, and encourages mobility.

- Social worker counsels and finds resources for clients.

Nursing Assistant/Nurse Aide Flash Review

FACTORS THAT AFFECT REHABILITATION

. . . .

ASSISTIVE DEVICES

. . . .

BOWEL AND BLADDER REHABILITATION

PART 6

- the client's age
- the client's overall health status
- the client's attitude
- the client's coping abilities
- the family's response to the client's disability

. . . .

Assistive devices help clients with their ADLs. These include devices to make eating easier, such as easy-grip mugs, utensils with easy-grip handles, utensil holders, and a food guard that attaches to the plate to make scooping food easier.

. . . .

Bowel and bladder rehabilitation is used for incontinent clients to enable them to regain full or partial control of their elimination patterns. The program includes adequate fluid intake, a high-fiber diet, and increased activity, as well as logging activities to determine voiding and defecating patterns.

NURSING ASSISTANT ROLE IN REHABILITATION

. . . .

URGENT PROBLEMS FOR REHABILITATION CLIENTS

. . . .

PART 6

The nursing assistant becomes the "eyes and ears" of the rehabilitation team. The nursing assistant's role in rehabilitation and restorative care includes the following:

- Learn how to care for client's specific rehabilitation needs, including the use of adaptive devices.
- Encourage client to practice the skills that are being learned.
- Assist client with bathing, dressing, and feeding.
- Assist client with using assistive devices.
- Assist with bowel and bladder retraining.
- Monitor the client's emotional status.
- Praise client for successes.
- Give client adequate time to complete tasks.
- Be empathetic.
- Seek support and guidance if frustrated with a client.

• •

When working with clients in rehabilitation, the nursing assistant should report the following client problems:

- thoughts of suicide
- signs of depression
- excessive difficulty with a new rehabilitative treatment
- pain, swelling, or redness near a supportive or prosthetic device
- supportive or adaptive device that is not working

• •

Nursing Assistant/Nurse Aide Flash Review

HOME HEALTHCARE

. . . .

CASE MANAGER

. . . .

HOME HEALTH AIDE

Home healthcare is the general term for a variety of health services that are performed in the client's home. Clients may receive home healthcare for a number of reasons, including:

• need for further care after hospital discharge

• chronic illness or disability that requires assistance

• illness that makes it dangerous for client to be alone

• terminal illness

· ·

The case manager is usually a registered nurse who oversees client care from admission through discharge.

· ·

Home health aides provide routine individualized healthcare to elderly clients, convalescent clients, chronically ill clients, or persons with disabilities at the client's home or in a care facility. Qualities of a successful home health aide include ability to work independently, be organized, manage time, be reliable, be resourceful, and set professional boundaries.

HOME HEALTH AIDE RESPONSIBILITIES

. . . .

RESPITE CARE

. . . .

Home health aide responsibilities may include:

- personal care: dressing, bathing, toileting, transferring
- utilizing items in the client's home when medical equipment is not available (e.g., using pillows to position client in semi-Fowler's position when there is no hospital bed)
- meal preparation
- light housekeeping
- assisting with infant care, including preparing formula

The home health aide should also be alert for safety hazards in the home and know how to get help in case of an emergency, and should contact the case manager for the following:

- changes in the client's level of consciousness or orientation
- changes or abnormalities in vital signs
- fever or other signs of infection
- skin breakdown or pressure ulcers
- signs of abuse
- unsanitary or unsafe conditions in the home

· ·

Respite care is short-term care given to a chronically ill or disabled client by another caregiver, so that a family member or friend who is the client's primary caregiver can rest and take time off. The goal is to decrease stress in primary caregivers while still filling the needs of the client who is receiving care.

· ·

NOTES

NOTES

NOTES

NOTES

NOTES